T0228930

Obstetric Ultrasound

Editor

EVA K. PRESSMAN

ULTRASOUND CLINICS

www.ultrasound.theclinics.com

Consulting Editor
VIKRAM DOGRA

January 2013 • Volume 8 • Number 1

ELSEVIER

1600 John F. Kennedy Boulevard • Suite 1800 • Philadelphia, Pennsylvania 19103-2899

http://www.theclinics.com

ULTRASOUND CLINICS Volume 8, Number 1
January 2013 ISSN 1556-858X, ISBN-13: 978-1-4557-7341-1

Editor: Donald Mumford

Ultrasound Clinics (ISSN 1556-858X) is published quarterly by W.B. Saunders, 360 Park Avenue South, New York, NY 10010-1710. Months of publication are January, April, July, and October. Business and editorial offices: 1600 John F. Kennedy Boulevard, Suite 1800, Philadelphia, Pennsylvania 19103-2899. Accounting and circulation offices: 6277 Sea Harbor Drive, Orlando, FL 32887-4800. Periodicals postage paid at New York, NY, and additional mailing offices. Subscription prices are $243 per year for (US individuals), $297 per year for (US institutions), $139 per year for (US students and residents), $273 per year for (Canadian individuals), $332 per year for (Canadian institutions), $291 per year for (international individuals), $332 per year for (international institutions), and $139 per year for (Canadian and foreign students/residents). To receive student/resident rate, orders must be accompanied by name of affiliated institution, date of term, and the signature of program/residency coordinator on institution letterhead. Orders will be billed at individual rate until proof of status is received. Foreign air speed delivery is included in all Clinics subscription prices. All prices are subject to change without notice. **POSTMASTER:** Send address changes to *Ultrasound Clinics,* Elsevier Health Sciences Division, Subscription Customer Service, 3251 Riverport Lane, Maryland Heights, MO 63043. **Customer Service (orders, claims, online, change of address): Telephone: 1-800-654-2452 (U.S. and Canada); 314-447-8871 (outside U.S. and Canada). Fax: 314-447-8029. E-mail: journalscustomerservice-usa@elsevier.com (for print support); journalsonlinesupport-usa@elsevier.com (for online support).**

Reprints: For copies of 100 or more, of articles in this publication, please contact the Commercial Reprints Department, Elsevier Inc., 360 Park Avenue South, New York, NY 10010-1710. Tel.: (+1) 212-633-3812; Fax: (+1) 212-462-1935; E-mail: reprints@elsevier.com.

Printed and bound by CPI Group (UK) Ltd, Croydon, CR0 4YY

Transferred to digital print 2012

Contributors

CONSULTING EDITOR

VIKRAM DOGRA, MD
Professor of Radiology, Urology, and Biomedical Engineering, Director of Ultrasound and Associate Chair for Education and Research, Department of Imaging Sciences, University of Rochester School of Medicine and Dentistry, Rochester, New York

GUEST EDITOR

EVA K. PRESSMAN, MD
Director of Maternal Fetal Medicine; Professor of Obstetrics and Gynecology, Department of Obstetrics and Gynecology, University of Rochester Medical Center, Rochester, New York

AUTHORS

ELIZABETH A. FOUNTAINE, MD
Obstetrics and Gynecology Resident, Department of Obstetrics and Gynecology, University of Rochester, Rochester, New York

DZHAMALA GILMANDYAR, MD
Maternal Fetal Medicine Fellow, Department of Obstetrics and Gynecology, University of Rochester School of Medicine, Rochester, New York

DAVID N. HACKNEY, MD, MS
Assistant Professor, Maternal Fetal Medicine, Department of Obstetrics and Gynecology, University of Rochester Medical Center, Rochester, New York

MONIQUE HO, MD
Assistant Professor of OB/GYN and Pediatrics, Director of Reproductive Genetics, Division of Maternal-Fetal Medicine, Department of OB/GYN, University of Rochester Medical Center, Rochester, New York

KRISTIN M. KNIGHT, MD, FACOG
Perinatologist, Maternal-Fetal Medicine Associates of Maryland, Rockville, Maryland

COURTNEY OLSON-CHEN, MD
Resident, Department of Obstetrics and Gynecology, University of Rochester Medical Center, Rochester, New York

TULIN OZCAN, MD
Associate Professor of Obstetrics and Gynecology, Department of Obstetrics and Gynecology, Rochester, New York

EVA K. PRESSMAN, MD
James R. Woods Professor of Obstetrics and Gynecology, Director of Maternal Fetal Medicine, Department of Obstetrics and Gynecology, University of Rochester Medical Center, Rochester, New York

NEIL S. SELIGMAN, MD, MS
Assistant professor, Division of Maternal-Fetal Medicine, Strong Memorial Hospital, University of Rochester, Rochester, New York

LORALEI L. THORNBURG, MD
Assistant Professor of OB/GYN, Division of Maternal Fetal Medicine, Department of OB/GYN, University of Rochester Medical Center, University of Rochester, Rochester, New York

PAULA ZOZZARO-SMITH, DO
Division of Maternal Fetal Medicine, Department of Obstetrics and Gynecology, University of Rochester, Rochester, New York

Contents

Preface ix

Eva K. Pressman

Ultrasound for Cervical Length 1

Courtney Olson-Chen and David N. Hackney

Cervical length can be a useful predictor of pregnancy outcomes, such as preterm birth. Transvaginal ultrasonography is a reproducible method for the evaluation of cervical length. This imaging examination is now used to assist in the triage and management of high-risk and symptomatic patients in addition to routine screening of asymptomatic pregnant women. The purpose of this article is to review the methods for cervical length measurement and discuss the implications of a short cervix. The information will be valuable in determining when to use cervical length measurement for screening and how to manage patients with a short cervix.

Ultrasound for Fetal Ventriculomegaly 13

Neil S. Seligman

Investigation of the fetal cerebral ventricle by ultrasound is currently recommended as part of the basic fetal ultrasound. Ventriculomegaly (VM) is among the most common central nervous system anomalies. Causes of VM include idiopathic causes, aneuploidy, genetic syndromes, viral infections, and central nervous system processes. Referral may be necessary for additional evaluation. Approximately 40% of fetuses with VM will be found to have associated cranial and extracranial anomalies. Fetuses with VM are at risk for miscarriage, stillbirth, neonatal/infant death, and abnormal long-term neurodevelopmental outcome. When an underlying etiology can be determined, the specific cause will determine the outcome.

Ultrasonography for Cesarean Scar Ectopics 27

Dzhamala Gilmandyar

The incidence of cesarean scar ectopic pregnancies is thought to have increased over the last decade. While still a rare occurrence, it is common enough that most obstetrics and gynecology providers should be familiar with various modes of evaluation and diagnosis. Transvaginal ultrasonography has proven irreplaceable in early diagnosis and subsequent evaluation of treatment response. This article reviews methods and techniques of sonographic diagnosis of this life-threatening condition.

Evaluation of Suspected Fetal Skeletal Dysplasia for the Referring Physician 31

Monique Ho

This article presents an overview of the presenting features of skeletal dysplasias commonly diagnosed in the fetus. An initial approach to prenatal evaluation of suspected skeletal dysplasia for the referring ultrasound practitioner is discussed.

Effects of Obesity on Obstetric Ultrasound Imaging 39

Loralei L. Thornburg

This article updates the obstetric community on the limitation of ultrasound scan in the obese patient, and the data regarding optimizing ultrasound care for this population. Special attention is given to the limitations of ultrasound scan for performing first-trimester genetic screening, genetic ultrasound scan, and anatomic evaluation and the limitations of ultrasound scan to predict birth weight in the obese patient.

Ultrasonography for Fetal Lung Masses 49

Paula Zozzaro-Smith

This article presents an overview of the most common fetal congenital lung masses identified by prenatal ultrasonography. Prenatal diagnosis, management, complications, and prognosis are reviewed.

Ultrasound for Abdominal Wall Defects 55 

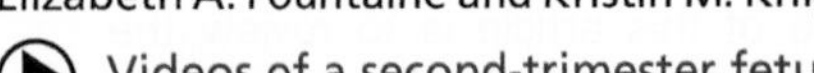
Elizabeth A. Fountaine and Kristin M. Knight

 Videos of a second-trimester fetus with gastroschisis accompany this article.

Abdominal wall defects are common congenital malformations diagnosed prenatally by ultrasound. This article reviews the most common forms of abdominal wall defects and describes how to differentiate between them ultrasonographically.

Ultrasonography for Fetal Hydronephrosis 69

Tulin Ozcan

Fetal hydronephrosis is a common problem on antenatal ultrasonography. This article summarizes the incidence, diagnosis, and management of fetal hydronephrosis.

Ultrasound for Evaluation of Fetal Anemia 79

Eva K. Pressman

 Video of transfusion into the placental insertion of the umbilical vein with an anterior placenta accompanies this article.

The management of fetal anemia remains one of the great success stories of intrauterine treatment. Advances in the diagnosis and treatment of fetal anemia are primarily related to advances in ultrasound resolution and the ability to safely perform ultrasound-guided fetal procedures. Management of fetal anemia relies on appropriate suspicion based on clinical history or sonographic findings, application of both invasive and noninvasive diagnostic technologies, and a combination of in utero therapy, delivery planning, and postnatal management. Noninvasive diagnosis of fetal anemia with Doppler velocimetry of the fetal middle cerebral artery has allowed better screening and earlier and more effective treatment.

Training for Ultrasound Procedures 89

Loralei L. Thornburg

 Videos on amniocentesis approach, term amniocentesis, transabdominal CVS, and transcervical CVS accompany this article.

This article provides an update on the training related to procedures performed during pregnancy, including amniocentesis, chorionic villus sampling, and fetal blood sampling. This information is of benefit to clinician educators and fellows as they teach and train in ultrasound-based procedures and for practicing clinicians to aid in training sonographers to assist during procedures.

Index 105

ULTRASOUND CLINICS

FORTHCOMING ISSUES

April 2013
Interventional Ultrasound
David Waldman, MD, *Guest Editor*

July 2013
Pediatric Ultrasound
Harriet Paltiel, MD, *Guest Editor*

October 2013
Genitourinary Ultrasound
Lorenzo Derchi, MD, *Guest Editor*

RECENT ISSUES

October 2012
Musculoskeletal Ultrasound
Diana Gaitini, MD, *Guest Editor*

July 2012
Ultrasound-Guided Procedures
Wael Saad, MBBCh, *Guest Editor*

April 2012
Head and Neck Ultrasound
Joseph C. Sniezek, MD, and
Robert A. Sofferman, MD, *Guest Editors*

RELATED INTEREST

December 2011
Obstetrics and Gynecology Clinics of North America
Advances in Laparoscopy and Minimally Invasive Surgery
Michael P. Traynor, MD, MPH, *Guest Editor*

PROGRAM OBJECTIVE:

The goal of the *Ultrasound Clinics* is to keep practicing radiologists and radiology residents up to date with current clinical practice in ultrasound by providing timely articles reviewing the state of the art in patient care.

TARGET AUDIENCE

Practicing radiologists, radiology residents and other healthcare professionals who provide care based on radiologic findings.

ACCREDITATION

The Elsevier Office of Continuing Medical Education (EOCME) is accredited by the Accreditation Council for Continuing Medical Education (ACCME) to provide continuing medical education for physicians.

The EOCME designates this journal-based CME activity for a maximum of 10 *AMA PRA Category 1 Credit*(s)™. Physicians should claim only the credit commensurate with the extent of their participation in the activity.

All other health care professionals completing continuing education credit for this activity will be issued a certificate of participation.

DISCLOSURE OF CONFLICTS OF INTEREST

The EOCME assesses conflict of interest with its instructors, faculty, planners, and other individuals who are in a position to control the content of CME activities. All relevant conflicts of interest that are identified are thoroughly vetted by EOCME for fair balance, scientific objectivity, and patient care recommendations. EOCME is committed to providing its learners with CME activities that promote improvements or quality in healthcare and not a specific proprietary business or a commercial interest.

The planning committee, staff, authors and editors listed below have identified no financial relationships or relationships to products or devices they or their spouse/life partner have with commercial interest related to the content of this CME activity:

Stephanie Carter; Elizabeth A. Fountaine, MD; David N. Hackney, MD, MS; Monique Ho, MD; Kristin M. Knight, MD, FACOG; Mahendra Kumar Chandran; Jill McNair; Courtney Olson-Chen, MD; Tulin Ozcan, MD; Eva K. Pressman, MD; Neil S. Seligman, MD, MS; Katelynn Steck; Loralei L. Thornburg, MD; and Paula Zozzaro-Smith, DO.

The planning committee, staff, authors and editors listed below have identified financial relationships or relationships to products or devices they or their spouse/life partner have with commercial interest related to the content of this CME activity:

Dzhamala Gilmandyar, MD has a spouse that works at Pfizer.

UNAPPROVED/OFF-LABEL USE DISCLOSURE

The EOCME requires CME faculty to disclose to the participants:

1. When products or procedures being discussed are off-label, unlabelled, experimental, and/or investigational (not US Food and Drug Administration [FDA]) approved; and
2. Any limitations on the information presented, such as data that are preliminary or that represent ongoing research, interim analyses, and/or unsupported opinions. Faculty may discuss information about pharmaceutical agents that is outside of DA-approved labelling. This information is intended solely for CME and is not intended to promote off-label use of these medications. If you have any questions, contact the medical affairs department of the manufacturer for the most recent prescribing information.

TO ENROLL

To enroll in the ***Ultrasounds Clinic*** Continuing Medical Education program, call customer service at 1-800-654-2452 or sign up online at **http://www.theclinics.com/home/cme**. The CME program is available to subscribers for an additional annual fee of $212.00.

METHOD OF PARTICIPATION

In order to claim credit, participants must complete the following:

1. Complete enrolment as indicated above.
2. Read the activity.
3. Complete the CME Test and Evaluation. Participants must achieve a score of 70% on the test. All CME Tests and Evaluations must be completed online.

CME INQUIRIES/SPECIAL NEEDS

For all CME inquiries or special needs, please contact elsevierCME@elsevier.com.

Preface

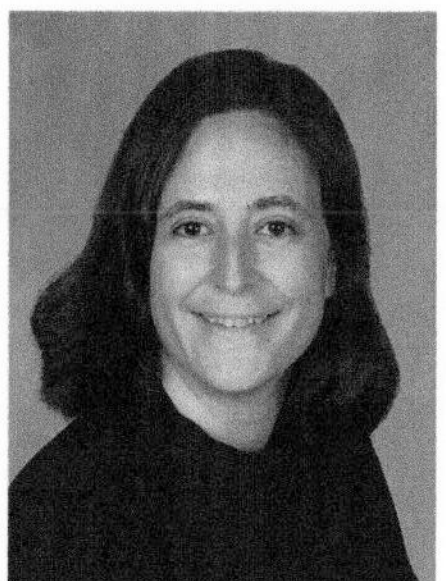

Eva K. Pressman, MD
Guest Editor

It has been a pleasure editing this issue of *Ultrasound Clinics* on selected topics in Obstetrics Ultrasound. The issue covers many of the challenges in prenatal diagnosis and obstetrical ultrasound evaluation and illuminates possible pitfalls and management considerations. In addition to covering complex fetal anomalies such as ventriculomegaly, skeletal dysplasias, fetal lung masses, abdominal wall defects, and hydronephrosis, this issue addresses the timely issues of sonographic assessment of cervical length, cesarean scar ectopics, evaluation for fetal anemia, and the effects of maternal obesity on obstetrical ultrasound imaging. In addition, at a time when the approach to fetal genetic diagnosis is rapidly changing and past approaches to training for ultrasound-guided procedures during pregnancy may no longer be practical, new approaches to training are described.

I wish to thank all of the authors for their thorough and timely reviews and the editorial staff at Elsevier for their help in putting this issue together. I hope that this issue will serve as a reference to all providers and trainees in the field of obstetrical ultrasound imaging.

Eva K. Pressman, MD
Department of Obstetrics and Gynecology
University of Rochester Medical Center
601 Elmwood Avenue
Rochester, NY 14642, USA

E-mail address:
eva_pressman@urmc.rochester.edu

Ultrasound Clin 8 (2013) ix
http://dx.doi.org/10.1016/j.cult.2012.09.002
1556-858X/13/$ – see front matter

Ultrasound for Cervical Length

Courtney Olson-Chen, MD[a], David N. Hackney, MD, MS[b,*]

KEYWORDS

• Cervical length • Short cervix • Preterm birth • Cerclage • Progesterone • Transvaginal ultrasound

KEY POINTS

- Transvaginal measurement of cervical length is one of the most effective methods for the prediction of preterm birth.
- The sensitivity of this screening test varies widely depending on the population.
- In all populations, the shorter the cervical length and the earlier it is detected in pregnancy, the higher the incidence of preterm birth.
- Interventions, including progesterone and cervical cerclage, can be used in these patients to greatly decrease the risk of preterm birth and subsequent neonatal morbidity and mortality.

HOW IS THE CERVICAL LENGTH MEASURED BY ULTRASOUND?

The length of a cervix can be evaluated either by sonogram or physical examination of the cervix. Digital examination has been shown to be less consistent than ultrasound in the assessment of cervical length.[1] The cervical length tends to be underestimated by manual examination by approximately 11 mm compared with ultrasound measurement.[2] In addition, physical changes like effacement are often not evident until the process is advanced; therefore, the absence of findings on physical examination cannot exclude a decreased cervical length.[3]

Sonographic measurement of cervical length can be performed by transabdominal, transvaginal, or transperineal examination.[3] The first imaging method used to measure cervical lengths was transabdominal ultrasonography.[4] A major disadvantage of transabdominal cervical length evaluation is the distortion caused by the bladder. If imaging is performed while patients have a full bladder, the cervical length can appear artificially lengthened.[5] The transabdominal view can also be obscured by maternal habitus, the position of the cervix, and the fetal presenting part.[6]

Transperineal ultrasonography is considered a reasonable alternative to transvaginal ultrasonography for measuring cervical length.[7] Transperineal evaluation of the cervical length was performed before the development of transvaginal transducers and may be useful when transvaginal ultrasonography is contraindicated. The transperineal probe is placed over the labia minora and aimed in the direction of the vaginal canal toward the cervix. Although this method of imaging correlates well with the transvaginal method, it is operator dependent and the image can be distorted by shadowing from the pelvic bones and rectal gas.[8,9] For these reasons, failure to obtain a clear image on transperineal ultrasound has been reported in up to 30% of cases.[9] There is conflicting evidence regarding patient preference of transvaginal versus transperineal ultrasound.[9,10] Transperineal

Disclosures: The authors have identified no professional or financial affiliations for themselves or their spouse/partner.

[a] Department of Obstetrics and Gynecology, University of Rochester Medical Center, 601 Elmwood Avenue, Rochester, NY 14642, USA; [b] Maternal Fetal Medicine, Department of Obstetrics and Gynecology, University of Rochester Medical Center, 601 Elmwood Avenue, Rochester, NY 14642, USA

* Corresponding author. Department of Obstetrics and Gynecology, University of Rochester Medical Center, School of Medicine and Dentistry, 601 Elmwood Avenue, Box 668, Rochester, NY 14642.

E-mail address: dnhackney@hotmail.com

Ultrasound Clin 8 (2013) 1–11
http://dx.doi.org/10.1016/j.cult.2012.08.010

sonography is also technically more difficult to perform.[11]

Transvaginal sonography has become the gold standard for measuring cervical length. It offers similar benefits as transperineal ultrasound in addition to improved visualization and decreased bowel gas artifact.[11] A recent study comparing transabdominal and transvaginal cervical lengths found that transabdominal measurement overestimated the cervical length by 8 mm in women with a short cervix, with only 43% of women with a short cervix being correctly diagnosed by transabdominal ultrasound.[12] Other studies have shown that transabdominal ultrasound tends to underestimate cervical length.[13] Given the unreliability of transabdominal measurement, transvaginal ultrasonography has emerged as the preferred method for the evaluation of cervical length. Transvaginal cervical imaging has minimal interobserver and intraobserver variability when performed correctly or according to a standardized protocol.[1,14] Accurate measurement of cervical length requires appropriate technique as described in **Box 1**,[11,15] and an example of a properly measured cervical length is provided in **Fig. 1**.

There are several anatomic and technical challenges of transvaginal ultrasonography to be cognizant of when measuring cervical length.[14,16] It can be difficult to consistently identify the internal os of the cervix secondary to uterine contractions and the dynamic nature of the cervix.[16] Past studies suggest waiting 3 to 5 minutes to detect changes in cervical length and shape.[17,18] Both the average of multiple measurements or the shortest measurement has been described. The shortest cervical length has the best predictive value related to the risk of preterm birth, and this is most often used as a standard for measurement.[18,19] Of note, if the cervical canal is curved, the measurement can be obtained by either tracing the cervical canal or using the sum of 2 straight lines that essentially follow the curve of the cervix. A curved cervix is defined by a deviation of greater than 5 mm from a straight line between the external and internal cervical os.[20] In general, if a cervix is curved, it is unlikely to be short.[15]

There may be distortion in transvaginal ultrasonography from the local anatomy, such as a large endocervical polyp.[16] Excessive pressure with the transvaginal probe on the anterior lip of the cervix can artificially elongate the cervical canal.[21] To avoid excess pressure, Burger and colleagues[21] recommend that the sonographer identify equal distances from the cervical canal to both the surface of the posterior lip and the surface of the anterior lip. Excessive pressure from the transvaginal probe will also often result in different echotextures between the anterior and posterior cervical lips. An example of a cervical length in which excessive pressure has been applied is provided in **Fig. 2**. Another common pitfall is the incorrect interpretation of an unusually thickened or echolucent endocervix as either cervical dilation or a funnel, as demonstrated in **Fig. 3**. An echolucent endocervical canal will usually be of a relatively uniform diameter throughout the length of the cervix, have a T-shaped internal os, and remain stable with the application of fundal pressure. A dilated or funneled cervix, by contrast, will often be more variable in appearance both along the length of the cervix and with the application of pressure. If one cannot clearly differentiate between the two entities sonographically, then

Box 1
Standardized measurement of transvaginal cervical length

1. Have the patient empty her bladder.
2. Cover the clean probe with a condom.
3. Insert the probe (or the patient can insert if desired).
4. Place the probe in the anterior fornix of the vagina.
5. Obtain a sagittal view of the cervix showing the long-axis view of echogenic endocervical mucosa along the length of the canal.
6. Withdraw the probe until the image becomes blurred, and then reapply just enough pressure to restore the image.
7. Enlarge the image until the cervix occupies at least two-thirds of the image and the internal and external os are well seen.
8. Measure the cervical length from the internal to the external os along the endocervical canal.
9. Obtain at least 3 measurements and record the shortest measurement.
10. Apply transfundal pressure for 15 seconds and measure the cervical length again at least 3 times.
11. The examination should last at least 5 minutes. Record only the shortest measurement for clinical management.

Adapted from Sonek JD, Iams JD, Blumenfeld M, et al. Measurement of cervical length in pregnancy: comparison between vaginal ultrasonography and digital examination; and Grimes-Dennis J, Berghella V. Cervical length and prediction of preterm delivery. Curr Opin Obstet Gynecol 2007;19:191–5.

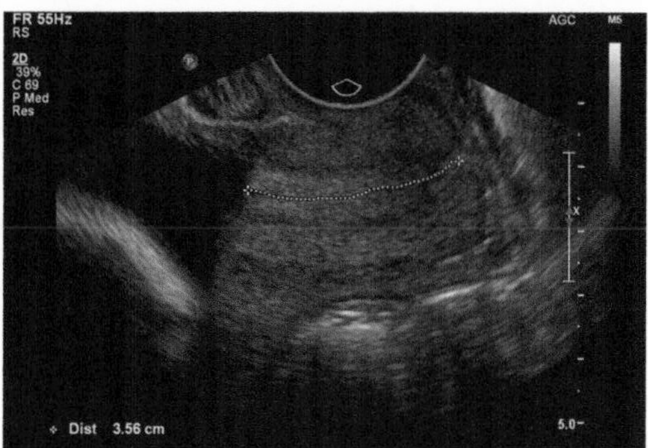

Fig. 1. Appropriately measured cervical length (*dotted line*).

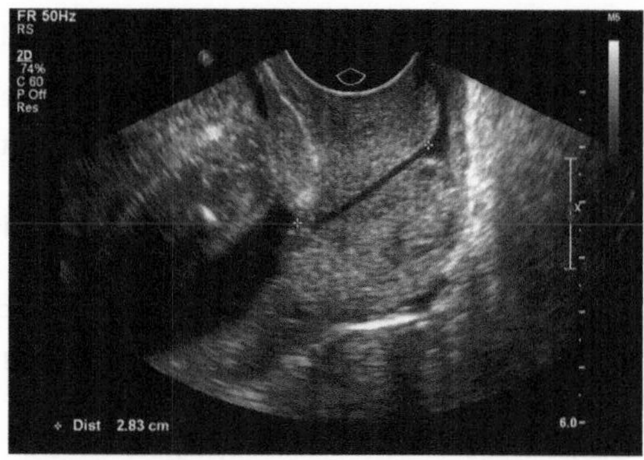

Fig. 3. Cervix with unusually echolucent cervical canal. The cervix remained stable with fundal pressure, was closed on digital examination, and remained stable on follow-up sonography.

a digital cervical examination could be performed, as well as a repeat ultrasound to ensure stability.

Both the American Congress of Obstetricians and Gynecologists (ACOG) and the American Institute of Ultrasound in Medicine recommend that the cervix be examined sonographically when feasible. They recommend that transvaginal or transperineal ultrasound be considered if the cervix appears shortened and cannot be adequately visualized with the transabdominal probe.[22,23] Many trials that include the measurement of cervical lengths require that the study sonographers participate in a training program to obtain certification in the transvaginal ultrasound of the cervix. When the appropriate views and measurements are examined as outlined in **Boxes 1** and **2**, the interobserver variation ranges from 5% to 10%.[1]

Funneling can also be evaluated by transvaginal ultrasound. This funneling occurs when the internal os of the cervix is opened. U-shaped funnels indicate preterm birth risk.[14] Care must be taken not to mistake a lower uterine segment contraction for funneling of the internal cervical os. This distinction should be resolved by performing the transvaginal ultrasound over 5 minutes.[15] Funneling may also be concealed with excessive probe pressure on the cervix or if the bladder is not empty. Importantly, funneling has higher interobserver variability among trained sonographers than cervical length measurement.[17] Fundal pressure during transvaginal ultrasound of the cervix may be useful for some patients.[15,24] The cervix can decrease in length in response to transfundal pressure approximately 5% of the time. It is unclear if fundal pressure increases the predictive accuracy of transvaginal ultrasound. There are specific requirements listed in **Box 2** for transvaginal imaging of cervical length that help to decrease error.[15]

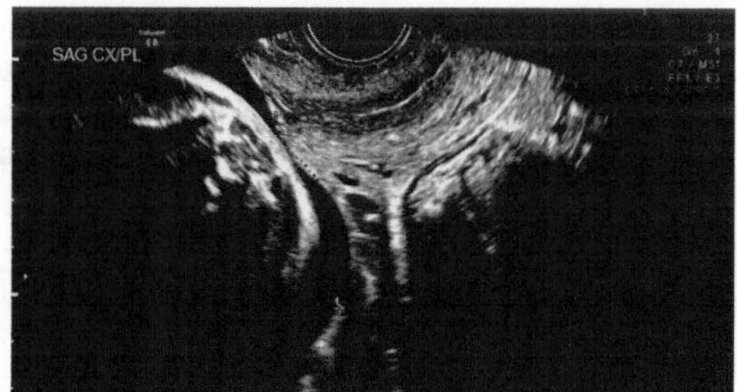

Fig. 2. Cervix with the application of excessive probe pressure. The anterior and posterior lip of the cervix differ in both thickness and echogenicity. The yellow line is an incidentally measured distance between the cervix and placenta.

Box 2
Requirements for transvaginal ultrasound

1. The internal os should be either flat or at an isosceles angle with regard to the uterus.
2. The length of the cervix should be visualized.
3. A symmetric image of the external os should be obtained.
4. The distance from the surface of the posterior lip to the cervical canal should be equal to the distance from the surface of the anterior lip to the cervical canal.
5. There should be no echogenicity in the cervix because this is a sign of excess pressure.

Adapted from Sonek JD, Iams JD, Blumenfeld M, et al. Measurement of cervical length in pregnancy: comparison between vaginal ultrasonography and digital examination. Obstet Gynecol 1990;76:172–5

Key points: ultrasound measurement of cervical length

- Digital examination underestimates cervical length compared with ultrasound measurement.
- Transabdominal measurement of cervical length can be obscured by the bladder, maternal habitus, or the presenting fetal part.
- Transperineal measurement of cervical length is operator dependent and can be distorted by shadowing from the pelvic bones and rectal gas.
- Transvaginal sonography has become the gold standard for measuring cervical length.
- The shortest cervical length measured transvaginally has the best predictive value related to the risk of preterm birth.
- When using a transvaginal probe, care should be taken to avoid excessive pressure on the cervix and to distinguish an echolucent endocervix from funneling.

WHEN IN PREGNANCY SHOULD THE CERVICAL LENGTH BE MEASURED?

Standards for the most optimal timing and frequency of cervical length measurements for screening have not been established. This lack of standardization is partly because many of the studies that have evaluated various interventions for decreased cervical lengths, such as vaginal progesterone or cerclage, have used differing screening protocols.[25–27] An intervention using cerclage for the prevention of preterm birth in women with a short cervix began measuring cervical length by ultrasound at 16 weeks' gestation, and no measurements were taken after 22 weeks' and 6 days' gestation.[25] Fonseca and colleagues[26] studied the use of vaginal progesterone in women with short cervical lengths measured between 20 and 25 weeks' gestation. Finally, another study investigating the use of vaginal progesterone used a screening protocol including women from 19 weeks' to 23 weeks' and 6 days' gestation.[27]

There is uncertainty regarding the earliest gestational age at which transvaginal imaging is beneficial. It can be difficult to differentiate the lower uterine segment from the endocervical canal in patients before 14 weeks' gestation. The gestational sac at this gestational age is not large enough to expand the lower uterine segment. Thus, many experts do not recommend measuring the cervical length before 14 weeks.[11]

With regard to an upper gestational age limit, a useful guiding principle is that one should not perform a test if the results would not lead to a change in patient management. Thus, the upper gestational age at which transvaginal ultrasound measurements of cervical length should be performed would be the age beyond which one would not intervene for a decreased length. For patients with active preterm labor symptoms who are undergoing a triage evaluation, the gestational age limit would be that for which one would intervene for the preterm labor itself. For asymptomatic patients, 2 of the more common interventions are cervical cerclage and vaginal progesterone. Cerclage is not usually used beyond the point of fetal viability, which in developed countries is usually 24 weeks. Likewise, 25 weeks is the highest gestational age at which patients have been enrolled in a large randomized controlled trial of vaginal progesterone.[26] Thus, there is no support for cervical length measurements beyond 25 weeks for these interventions. Beyond 25 weeks, one could hypothetically use cervical length measurements to guide the use of bed rest, work or activity restrictions, or the prophylactic use of steroids for fetal pulmonary maturity, although the utility of these interventions in asymptomatic patients is not clear. Although variation exists among practitioners in this regard, it is not the practice of these authors to perform transvaginal ultrasound measurements in asymptomatic patients beyond 25 weeks.

Key points: timing of cervical length measurement

- There is no standard for the most optimal timing and frequency of cervical length measurements.
- Experts do not recommend measuring cervical length before 14 weeks because it can be difficult to differentiate the lower uterine segment from the endocervical canal.
- The upper gestational age limit for measurement of cervical length is the age at which one would not intervene for a shortened cervix.

Key points: implications of a decreased cervical length

- The preterm birth rate in the United States is 11.99%, and preterm birth leads to significant perinatal morbidity and mortality.
- The incidence of spontaneous preterm birth increases as the cervical length decreases.
- However, most women (75%) with short cervices do not deliver preterm.
- Transvaginal ultrasound measurement of cervical length is best as a predictor of preterm birth in singleton gestations and women with an increased risk of preterm birth.

WHAT ARE THE IMPLICATIONS OF A DECREASED CERVICAL LENGTH?

Preterm birth remains a leading cause of perinatal morbidity and mortality worldwide. The preterm birth rate in the United States is 11.99% based on vital records from 2010.[28] Most preterm births are caused by preterm labor with or without the premature rupture of membranes. Although most of these infants survive, they have an increased prevalence of neurodevelopmental impairments and respiratory complications.[29] Costs of preterm birth admissions totaled $5.8 billion in 2001. These costs were highest for extremely premature infants, or those less than 28 weeks' gestation, with an average of $65 600 per infant.[30] The identification of risk factors for preterm birth is, therefore, an important challenge currently under investigation. Early prediction of an outcome like preterm birth allows time for interventions.

Transvaginal sonography of cervical length could have a major clinical impact in the identification of patients at risk for preterm birth. In a large prospective multicenter study, Iams and colleagues[17] found that the incidence of spontaneous preterm birth increased as the cervical length at 24 to 28 weeks' gestation decreased. The 10th percentile had a cervical length of less than 25 mm. Therefore, this measurement is commonly used as the threshold to define a short cervix. The risk of preterm delivery continued to increase at cervical lengths even more than the 10th percentile. For example, women with cervical lengths at or less than the 75th percentile had a significantly increased risk of preterm delivery compared with those with cervical lengths greater than the 75th percentile. The data from this study suggest that cervical length should be seen as a continuous, not dichotomous, variable.[17] Although a clear relationship between a shortened cervix on transvaginal ultrasound and preterm birth has been established, it is important to remember that most women (75%) with shortened cervices do not deliver preterm.[17] Hence, decreased cervical lengths have a much higher negative predictive value than positive predictive value (**Fig. 4**).

Transvaginal ultrasound is best as a predictor of preterm birth in singleton gestations. The sensitivity of this measurement is much higher in singleton gestations compared with multiple gestations because multiples with preterm birth often do not have a short cervical length during the second trimester.[31] Transvaginal ultrasound is also more sensitive (>50%) in women with an increased risk of preterm birth, which includes women with a history of preterm birth, previous cone biopsy, or Mullerian anomaly. On the other hand, transvaginal cervical length measurement in women with no risk factors for preterm birth has a sensitivity of only 37%.[17] The following sections address the management of shortened cervix in various patient scenarios.

PATIENTS WITH A HISTORY OF PRETERM BIRTH

Two of the primary potential interventions for patients with a history of a prior preterm birth

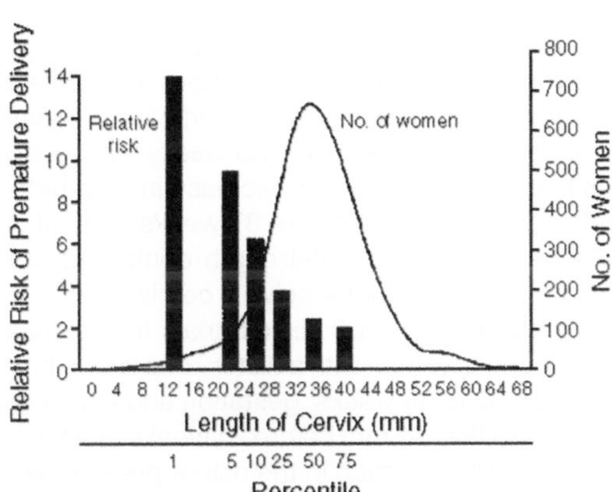

Fig. 4. Normal distribution of cervical length. (*Reprinted from* Iams JD, Goldenberg RL, Meis PJ, et al. The length of the cervix and the risk of spontaneous premature delivery. National Institute of Child Health and Human Development Maternal Fetal Medicine Unit Network. N Engl J Med 1996;334:567–72, Copyright © 1996, Massachusetts Medical Society; with permission.)

Key points: patients with a history of preterm birth

- The use of weekly intramuscular progesterone in patients with a history of a prior preterm birth leads to a decrease incidence of preterm birth.
- Cerclage can be considered in women with a history of preterm birth, a singleton gestation, and a cervical length less than 25 mm.

and a short cervical length are cervical cerclage and progesterone supplementation. With regard to progesterone supplementation, many patients will already be receiving this medication before the discovery of a short cervical length secondary to their preterm birth history alone. A randomized controlled trial performed by Meis and colleagues[32] demonstrated a decreased risk of preterm birth with the use of weekly intramuscular 17α-hydroxyprogesterone caproate in patients with a history of a prior preterm birth. Patients in this study received the progesterone secondary to their preterm birth history alone without additional stratification by cervical length. This finding was supported by a meta-analysis of multiple randomized trials.[33] ACOG recommends progesterone supplementation for the prevention of recurrent preterm birth in women with a singleton pregnancy and a prior spontaneous preterm birth.[34]

Owen and colleagues[25] evaluated the role of cerclage in women with a short cervix and history of preterm birth. This randomized trial monitored patients with serial transvaginal cervical lengths once every 2 weeks from 16 weeks' to 23 weeks' gestation. If the cervical length decreased to 25 to 30 mm, patients would return for weekly transvaginal ultrasounds. Women with a cervical length less than 25 mm were randomized to cerclage placement. No decrease in the primary outcome of preterm birth at less than 35 weeks was found, but there was a significant decrease in both births before 24 weeks and before 37 weeks in addition to a decrease in perinatal death compared with the group who did not receive a cerclage.[25]

A meta-analysis of 5 clinical trials for cerclage placement in women with a history of preterm birth less than 32 to 36 weeks' gestation and a cervical length less than 25 mm before 24 weeks' gestation found a 30% reduction in the risk of preterm birth less than 35 weeks' gestation and a 36% reduction in composite perinatal mortality and morbidity. This review concluded that cerclage prevents preterm birth specifically in women with a previous spontaneous preterm birth, singleton gestation, and cervical length less than 25 mm. The number needed to treat to prevent one recurrent preterm birth is 8. Of note, the use of cerclage does not apply to women with multiples, history of cervical surgery, or no history of preterm birth.[35]

PATIENTS WITH SYMPTOMS OF PRETERM LABOR

Many patients presenting with symptoms of preterm labor undergo prolonged observation and serial examinations to rule out cervical change. A more efficient method for identifying patients at a high risk of preterm birth would be helpful to optimize resources and begin early intervention while avoiding unnecessary treatment of women with a low risk of preterm birth. Examination of cervical length has been useful in predicting the risk of preterm birth in women presenting with symptoms of preterm labor. In one study, no patients with a cervical length more than 3 cm delivered within 21 days of the diagnosis of preterm labor.[8] The Ohio State University (OSU) Medical Center developed an early protocol for the management of patients presenting with concern for preterm labor (**Fig. 5**). The diagnosis of preterm labor is initially established if the cervix is 80% or more effaced or 3 cm or more dilated in the presence of regular contractions. If patients do not qualify as preterm labor by the preceding definition, a cervical length is performed. Preterm labor is considered very unlikely if the patients' cervix is 30 mm or more in length. Alternatively, patients with cervical lengths less than 20 mm and regular contractions are diagnosed with preterm labor. When the cervical length ranges from 20 to 30 mm, the OSU protocol recommends fetal fibronectin (FFN) testing. Those with positive FFN testing receive antenatal corticosteroids; if contractions occur 6 or more times per hour, they are treated with tocolysis. Preterm labor in the subsequent 14 days is considered very unlikely with a negative FFN. If ultrasound and FFN testing are not available, Guinn and colleagues[36] suggests the use of a single dose of subcutaneous terbutaline to identify women with symptoms in need of further evaluation.

Ness and colleagues,[37] at the Thomas Jefferson University Hospital, randomized patients with threatened preterm labor to management with

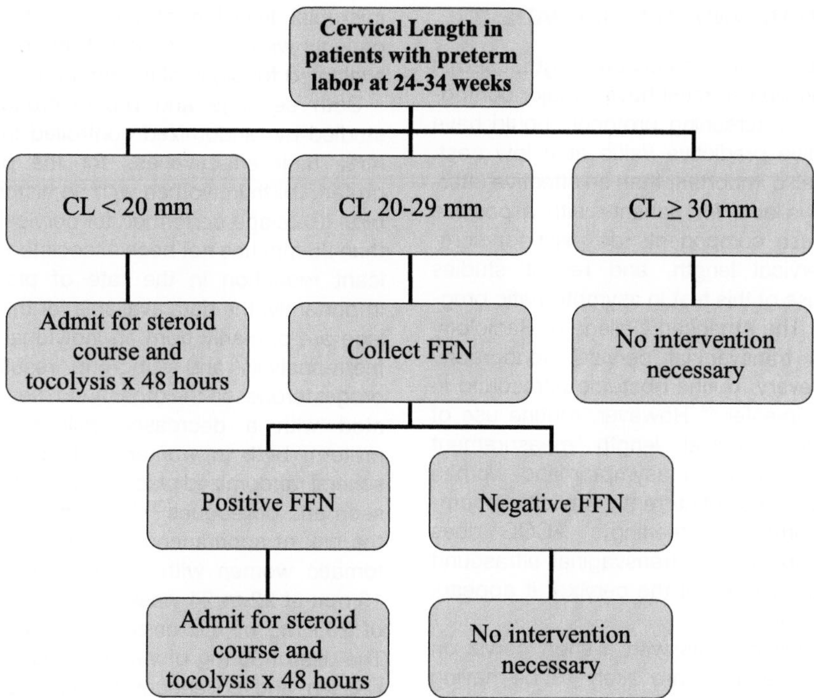

Fig. 5. Preterm labor protocol. CL, cervical length; FFN, fetal fibronectin. (*Data from* Berghella V, Bega G, Tolosa JE, et al. Ultrasound assessment of the cervix. Clin Obstet Gynecol 2003;46:947–62; and Ness A, Visintine J, Ricci E, et al. Does knowledge of cervical length and fetal fibronectin affect management of women with threatened preterm labor? A randomized trial. Am J Obstet Gynecol 2007;197:426.e1–7.)

the OSU protocol[38] versus a standard group without access to cervical length or fetal fibronectin testing. The study aimed to compare the length of evaluation in triage for these two groups. They found no significant difference between the groups in the length of evaluation. However, the mean time for evaluation was significantly shorter in the group following the OSU protocol specifically in women with a cervical length 30 mm or more. The knowledge of cervical length and FFN results was also associated with a decreased incidence of preterm birth. The study also noted that the addition of FFN results did not improve the positive predictive value of cervical lengths less than 20 mm.

Based on the findings of the Ness study while using the OSU protocol, Berghella and colleagues[15] stated that the flow chart outlined in **Fig. 3** can be used for management of symptomatic women with preterm labor between 24 and 34 weeks. Of note, the inclusion criteria used for implementing this management for preterm labor were 6 or more contractions per hour or symptoms suggestive of preterm labor, including cramping and pressure. Women should also be less than 3 cm dilated and less than 100% effaced with intact membranes.

Key points: patients with symptoms of preterm birth

- The measurement of cervical length can be used to triage patients with symptoms of preterm birth.
- Preterm labor is very unlikely if the patients' cervix is 30 mm or more in length.
- Patients with cervical lengths less than 20 mm and regular contractions are likely to be in true preterm labor.
- One protocol recommends FFN testing for further evaluation when the cervical length ranges from 20 to 30 mm.

ASYMPTOMATIC AND LOW-RISK PATIENTS

A screening test, such as cervical length, used in asymptomatic women must have 2 major components. First, the screening protocol should have a high negative predictive value at a low cost. Second, it is also important than an effective intervention be available for patients with a positive screen.[38] These components do exist for screening of cervical length, and recent studies support the use of this test in asymptomatic pregnant women. The American College of Radiology recommends transvaginal cervical sonography as a part of every routine obstetric ultrasound in the second trimester.[24] However, routine use of ultrasound for cervical length measurement remains controversial in asymptomatic women and the ACOG does not currently explicitly recommend this form of screening.[34] ACOG does recommend obtaining a transvaginal ultrasound for further assessment of the cervix if it appears short transabdominally.[22]

Asymptomatic patients with a short cervix on transvaginal ultrasound are likely to be having contractions that they do not recognize. Women at less than 28 weeks' gestation with a significantly shorted cervical length should be evaluated with tocometry to ensure that they are not having asymptomatic uterine contractions. The presence of contractions doubles the risk of preterm delivery in patients with a shortened cervix. The cervix should be digitally assessed in asymptomatic patients with a short cervix. A short cervix has also been associated with an increased risk of microbial invasion of the amniotic cavity, and patients with an incidental short cervix should be evaluated for signs of intrauterine infection.[39]

Both cerclage and progesterone have been studied by randomized controlled trials to determine their effectiveness for the prevention of preterm birth in women with no history of preterm birth. Cerclage performed for cervical lengths less than 25 mm has not been associated with a significant reduction in the rate of preterm birth.[40] Importantly, the data available for the use of cerclage are primarily from an individual patient data meta-analysis and subgroup results.[40] Vaginal progesterone, on the other hand, has been associated with a decreased risk of spontaneous preterm birth in women with a short cervix in several randomized placebo-controlled trials. Fonseca and colleagues[26] found a 44% decrease in the risk of spontaneous preterm birth in asymptomatic women with cervical lengths less than 15 mm at 22 to 24 weeks' gestation with the use of 200 mg of micronized vaginal progesterone. The use of 90 mg of vaginal progesterone gel by Hassan and colleagues[27] demonstrated a 45% decreased risk of spontaneous preterm birth in asymptomatic women with a cervical length of 10.o to 20.9 mm at 19 to 24 weeks' gestation.

A recent individual patient data meta-analysis evaluated 5 randomized controlled trials of vaginal progesterone for midtrimester shortened cervical length.[41] Although the studies varied in their inclusion criteria and progesterone dose (**Table 1**), the pooled results showed that vaginal progesterone significantly reduced the rate of preterm birth at

Table 1
Characteristics of trials included in the vaginal progesterone meta-analysis

Study	Target Population	Cervical Length Criteria	Vaginal Progesterone Dose	Progesterone Gestational Age	Primary Outcome
[a]Fonseca et al,[26] 2007	Short cervix	CL ≤15 mm	200 mg capsule	24–33 6/7 wk	PTB <34 wk
O'Brien et al,[42] 2007	History of PTB	CL ≤25 mm	90 mg gel	18–37 wk	PTB <32 wk
Cetingoz et al,[43] 2011	High risk of PTB	CL ≤25 mm	100 mg suppository	24–34 wk	PTB <37 wk
[a]Hassan et al,[27] 2011	Short cervix	CL 10–20 mm	90 mg gel	20–36 6/7 wk	PTB <33 wk
Rode et al,[44] 2011	Twin pregnancy	CL ≤25 mm	200 mg pessary	20–33 6/7 wk	PTB <34 wk

Abbreviations: CL, cervical length; PTB, preterm birth.
[a] Largest trials.
Data from Romero R, Nicolaides K, Conde-Agudelo A, et al. Vaginal progesterone in women with an asymptomatic sonographic short cervix in the midtrimester decreases preterm delivery and neonatal morbidity: a systematic review and metaanalysis of individual patient data. Am J Obstet Gynecol 2012;206:124.e1–19.

Key points: asymptomatic/low-risk patients

- Routine cervical length measurement remains controversial in asymptomatic women.
- ACOG recommends transvaginal measurement of cervical length if the cervix appears short transabdominally.
- Tocometry should be considered for patients with a short cervical length to evaluate for asymptomatic contractions.
- Cerclage has not been associated with a significant reduction in the rate of preterm birth in asymptomatic women with a shortened cervix in the absence of a history of prior preterm birth.
- Vaginal progesterone has been associated a decreased risk of spontaneous preterm birth in asymptomatic women with a cervix less than 20 mm in length.
- Universal transvaginal ultrasound screening for cervical length and treatment with vaginal progesterone is a cost-effective strategy for the prevention of preterm birth.
- Routine use of transvaginal ultrasound is accepted by most women.

less than 35 weeks', less than 33 weeks', and less than 28 weeks' gestation. Vaginal progesterone was also associated with a decreased risk of infant respiratory distress syndrome and composite neonatal morbidity and mortality. A benefit was found for both women with no previous preterm birth and those with a history of at least one prior spontaneous preterm birth. The study recommends that screening of asymptomatic cervical lengths be performed at 19 to 24 weeks' gestation. There is not enough information to recommend vaginal progesterone for cervical lengths more than 20 mm or short cervical lengths detected after 26 weeks' gestation.[41]

A cost-effectiveness analysis performed by Cahill and colleagues[45] reported that universal transvaginal ultrasound screening for cervical length and treatment with vaginal progesterone was the most cost-effective strategy for the prevention of preterm birth. This strategy was preferred over cervical length screening only in women at an increased risk for preterm birth, treatment with intramuscular progesterone without screening, or no screening. On average, universal sonographic screening of cervical length saved $1339 per patient. This savings is largely caused by the decrease in the number of preterm births with the use of progesterone in women with a shortened cervix.

Although the use of universal cervical length screening is still controversial, an effective intervention now exists with the use of progesterone to decrease the risk of preterm birth. Because only a small percentage of patients will have a decreased cervical length, a very large number of transvaginal ultrasounds would be performed with routine screening. However, this seems to still be cost-effective given the tremendous expenses associated with preterm birth. Routine transvaginal ultrasound may not be acceptable to all patients and it could lead to an increased medicalization of normal pregnancies. However, one study reported that transvaginal sonography was accepted by more than 99% of women, and less than 2% of women reported pain associated with this method of ultrasound.[46] If pregnant women are counseled regarding the role of transvaginal ultrasound in the prediction and prevention of preterm birth, they will likely be even more willing to undergo this examination.

FUTURE STUDIES

There are several unanswered questions related to cervical length in pregnancy that are in need of further investigation. For example, there is no definitive evidence to determine if progesterone and cervical cerclage have an additive benefit in decreasing the risk of preterm birth. In addition, insufficient information is available regarding the potential benefits of cervical length assessment for certain high-risk women, including those with a history of cervical surgical procedures and those with Mullerian anomalies. Finally, there is a great need to identify and evaluate other more effective interventions for the prevention of preterm birth in women with a shortened cervix.

SUMMARY

Transvaginal measurement of cervical length is one of the most effective methods for the prediction of preterm birth. Proper technique must be used as outlined in **Box 1** and **Fig. 1**. The sensitivity of this screening test varies widely depending on the population. However, in all populations, the shorter the cervical length and the earlier it is detected in pregnancy, the higher the incidence of preterm birth. Interventions, including progesterone and cervical cerclage, can be used in these patients to greatly decrease the risk of preterm birth and subsequent neonatal morbidity and mortality.

REFERENCES

1. Sonek JD, Iams JD, Blumenfeld M, et al. Measurement of cervical length in pregnancy: comparison between vaginal ultrasonography and digital examination. Obstet Gynecol 1990;76:172–5.
2. Grimes-Dennis J, Berghella V. Cervical length and prediction of preterm delivery. Curr Opin Obstet Gynecol 2007;19:191–5.
3. Berghella V, Kuhlman K, Weiner S, et al. Cervical funneling: sonographic criteria predictive of preterm delivery. Ultrasound Obstet Gynecol 1997;10:161–6.
4. Sarti DA, Sample WF, Hobel CJ, et al. Ultrasonic visualization of a dilated cervix during pregnancy. Radiology 1979;130:417–20.
5. Andersen HF. Transvaginal and transabdominal ultrasonography of the uterine cervix during pregnancy. J Clin Ultrasound 1991;19:77–83.
6. Confino E, Mayden KL, Giglia RV, et al. Pitfalls in sonographic imaging of the incompetent uterine cervix. Acta Obstet Gynecol Scand 1986;65:593–7.
7. Richey SD, Ramin KD, Roberts SW, et al. The correlation between transperineal sonography and digital examination in the evaluation of the third-trimester cervix. Obstet Gynecol 1995;85:745–8.
8. Benson CB, Bluth EI. Ultrasonography in obstetrics and gynecology: a practical approach to clinical problems. 2nd edition. New York: Thieme; 2008.
9. Meijer-Hoogeveen M, Stoutenbeek P, Visser GH. Transperineal versus transvaginal sonographic cervical length measurement in second- and third-trimester pregnancies. Ultrasound Obstet Gynecol 2008;32:657–62.
10. Cicero S, Skentou C, Souka A, et al. Cervical length at 22-24 weeks of gestation: comparison of transvaginal and transperineal-translabial ultrasonography. Ultrasound Obstet Gynecol 2001;17:335–40.
11. Berghella VB, Bega G. Ultrasound evaluation of the cervix. In: Callen PW, editor. 5th edition. Philadelphia: Saunders Elsevier; 2008. p. 698–720.
12. Hernandez-Andrade E, Romero R, Ahn H, et al. Transabdominal evaluation of uterine cervical length during pregnancy fails to identify a substantial number of women with a short cervix. J Matern Fetal Neonatal Med 2012;25(9):1682–9.
13. Stone PR, Chan EH, McCowan LM, et al. Transabdominal scanning of the cervix at the 20-week morphology scan: comparison with transvaginal cervical measurements in a healthy nulliparous population. Aust N Z J Obstet Gynaecol 2010;50:523–7.
14. Mella MT, Berghella V. Prediction of preterm birth: cervical sonography. Semin Perinatol 2009;33:317–24.
15. Berghella V, Bega G, Tolosa JE, et al. Ultrasound assessment of the cervix. Clin Obstet Gynecol 2003;46:947–62.
16. Yost NP, Bloom SL, Twickler DM, et al. Pitfalls in ultrasonic cervical length measurement for predicting preterm birth. Obstet Gynecol 1999;93:510–6.
17. Iams JD, Goldenberg RL, Meis PJ, et al. The length of the cervix and the risk of spontaneous premature delivery. National Institute of Child Health and Human Development Maternal Fetal Medicine Unit Network. N Engl J Med 1996;334:567–72.
18. Sonek J, Shellhaas C. Cervical sonography: a review. Ultrasound Obstet Gynecol 1998;11:71–8.
19. Jenkins SM, Kurtzman JT, Osann K. Dynamic cervical change: is real-time sonographic cervical shortening predictive of preterm delivery in patients with symptoms of preterm labor? Ultrasound Obstet Gynecol 2006;27:373–6.
20. Owen J, Yost N, Berghella V, et al. Mid-trimester endovaginal sonography in women at high risk for spontaneous preterm birth. JAMA 2001;286:1340–8.
21. Burger M, Weber-Rossler T, Willmann M. Measurement of the pregnant cervix by transvaginal sonography: an interobserver study and new standards to improve the interobserver variability. Ultrasound Obstet Gynecol 1997;9:188–93.
22. American College of Obstetricians and Gynecologists. ACOG practice bulletin no. 101: ultrasonography in pregnancy. Obstet Gynecol 2009;113:451–61.
23. Medicine AIoU. AIUM practice guideline for the performance of obstetric ultrasound examinations; 2007:1–11.
24. Imaging EPoWs. Assessment of the gravid cervix. Available at: http://www.acr.org/Quality-Safety/Appropriateness-Criteria/Diagnostic/Womens-Imaging. Accessed May 4, 2012.
25. Owen J, Hankins G, Iams JD, et al. Multicenter randomized trial of cerclage for preterm birth prevention in high-risk women with shortened midtrimester cervical length. Am J Obstet Gynecol 2009;201:375.e1–8.
26. Fonseca EB, Celik E, Parra M, et al. Progesterone and the risk of preterm birth among women with a short cervix. N Engl J Med 2007;357:462–9.
27. Hassan SS, Romero R, Vidyadhari D, et al. Vaginal progesterone reduces the rate of preterm birth in women with a sonographic short cervix: a multicenter, randomized, double-blind, placebo-controlled trial. Ultrasound Obstet Gynecol 2011;38:18–31.
28. Hamilton BE, Martin JA, Ventura SJ. Births: preliminary data for 2010. Natl Vital Stat Rep 2011;60:1–25.

29. Goldenberg RL, Culhane JF, Iams JD, et al. Epidemiology and causes of preterm birth. Lancet 2008; 371:75–84.
30. Russell RB, Green NS, Steiner CA, et al. Cost of hospitalization for preterm and low birth weight infants in the United States. Pediatrics 2007;120: e1–9.
31. Goldenberg RL, Iams JD, Miodovnik M, et al. The preterm prediction study: risk factors in twin gestations. National Institute of Child Health and Human Development Maternal-Fetal Medicine Units Network. Am J Obstet Gynecol 1996;175:1047–53.
32. Meis PJ, Klebanoff M, Thom E, et al. Prevention of recurrent preterm delivery by 17 alpha-hydroxyprogesterone caproate. N Engl J Med 2003;348:2379–85.
33. Rode L, Langhoff-Roos J, Andersson C, et al. Systematic review of progesterone for the prevention of preterm birth in singleton pregnancies. Acta Obstet Gynecol Scand 2009;88:1180–9.
34. Society for Maternal Fetal Medicine Publications Committee. ACOG committee opinion number 419 October 2008 (replaces no. 291, November 2003). Use of progesterone to reduce preterm birth. Obstet Gynecol 2008;112:963–5.
35. Berghella V, Rafael TJ, Szychowski JM, et al. Cerclage for short cervix on ultrasonography in women with singleton gestations and previous preterm birth: a meta-analysis. Obstet Gynecol 2011;117:663–71.
36. Guinn DA, Goepfert AR, Owen J, et al. Management options in women with preterm uterine contractions: a randomized clinical trial. Am J Obstet Gynecol 1997;177:814–8.
37. Ness A, Visintine J, Ricci E, et al. Does knowledge of cervical length and fetal fibronectin affect management of women with threatened preterm labor? A randomized trial. Am J Obstet Gynecol 2007;197:426.e1–7.
38. Iams JD. Prediction and early detection of preterm labor. Obstet Gynecol 2003;101:402–12.
39. Gomez R, Romero R, Nien JK, et al. A short cervix in women with preterm labor and intact membranes: a risk factor for microbial invasion of the amniotic cavity. Am J Obstet Gynecol 2005;192:678–89.
40. Berghella V, Odibo AO, To MS, et al. Cerclage for short cervix on ultrasonography: meta-analysis of trials using individual patient-level data. Obstet Gynecol 2005;106:181–9.
41. Romero R, Nicolaides K, Conde-Agudelo A, et al. Vaginal progesterone in women with an asymptomatic sonographic short cervix in the midtrimester decreases preterm delivery and neonatal morbidity: a systematic review and metaanalysis of individual patient data. Am J Obstet Gynecol 2012;206:124. e1–124.e19.
42. O'Brien JM, Adair CD, Lewis DF, et al. Progesterone vaginal gel for the reduction of recurrent preterm birth: primary results from a randomized, double-blind, placebo-controlled trial. Ultrasound Obstet Gynecol 2007;30:687–96.
43. Cetingoz E, Cam C, Sakalli M, et al. Progesterone effects on preterm birth in high-risk pregnancies: a randomized placebo-controlled trial. Arch Gynecol Obstet 2011;283:423–9.
44. Rode L, Klein K, Nicolaides KH, et al. Prevention of preterm delivery in twin gestations (PREDICT): a multicenter, randomized, placebo-controlled trial on the effect of vaginal micronized progesterone. Ultrasound Obstet Gynecol 2011;38:272–80.
45. Cahill AG, Odibo AO, Caughey AB, et al. Universal cervical length screening and treatment with vaginal progesterone to prevent preterm birth: a decision and economic analysis. Am J Obstet Gynecol 2010;202:548.e1–8.
46. Dutta RL, Economides DL. Patient acceptance of transvaginal sonography in the early pregnancy unit setting. Ultrasound Obstet Gynecol 2003;22: 503–7.

Ultrasound for Fetal Ventriculomegaly

Neil S. Seligman, MD, MS

KEYWORDS

- Fetal ventriculomegaly • Fetal hydrocephalus • Congenital anomalies
- Central nervous system anomalies

KEY POINTS

- Ventriculomegaly (VM), defined as an atrial width of at least 10 mm, is a relatively common fetal anomaly and among the most common central nervous system anomalies.
- Routine evaluation of the fetal cerebral ventricles is recommended as part of the basic fetal ultrasound.
- Systematic evaluation of the ventricles in the 2-dimensional transverse plane may reduce overestimation of atrial width and false-positive results, and improve reproducibility.
- VM can be idiopathic or due to chromosomal disorders, genetic syndromes, viral infections, other central nervous system processes (eg, spina bifida, agenesis of the corpus callosum).
- Isolated VM is associated with improved survival and neurodevelopmental outcome; a careful and timely evaluation is required to ensure a complete assessment.

In the fetus, enlargement of the lateral cerebral ventricles is referred to as ventriculomegaly (VM). VM is a sensitive indicator of anomalous brain development,[1] which may predict subsequent neurologic impairment; however, isolated, mild VM is often benign. It is a relatively common fetal anomaly in general, and among the most common anomalies of the fetal central nervous system. The exact incidence of VM is unclear, but estimates suggest an incidence ranging from 0.7 to 1.5 cases per 1000 births, with the lower estimates reflecting isolated cases.[2–7] McGahan and Phillips first investigated the fetal ventricular atrium by ultrasound in 1983.[8] Presently, evaluation of the lateral cerebral ventricles is routinely included in the basic fetal ultrasound.[9–11] Dilatation of the lateral ventricles includes a spectrum of conditions ranging from isolated, mild VM to hydrocephalus with associated anomalies.[12] The causes of VM are heterogeneous, including both nervous and non-nervous pathologic conditions.

WHAT IS THE DEFINITION OF CEREBRAL VM?

According to Hilpert and colleagues,[13] the pooled mean atrial diameter across 9 studies including 8216 fetuses was 6.4 mm with a standard deviation of 1.2 mm (10 mm = 3 standard deviations (SD) above the mean). In a more recent analysis of 5610 fetuses, the mean was 6.55 mm, with a standard deviation of 1.31 mm (10 mm = 2.63 SD).[14] The diameter of the ventricular atrium remains constant in the second and third trimesters, with a mean of 5.4 to 7.6 mm reported consistently in multiple studies.[2,3,12–21] The upper limit of normal, 10 mm, is 2.5 to 4 standard deviations above the mean.

VM is defined as enlargement of the cerebral ventricles greater than 10 mm measured as the transverse diameter of the atrium. The degree of VM can be classified based on atrial diameter as mild between 10 and 15 mm and severe greater than 15 mm (**Fig. 1**); however, some authors

Disclosures: No funding or conflicts of interest to declare.

Division of Maternal-Fetal Medicine, Strong Memorial Hospital, University of Rochester, 601 Elmwood Avenue, Box 668, Rochester, NY 14642, USA

E-mail address: neil_seligman@urmc.rochester.edu

Ultrasound Clin 8 (2013) 13–25
http://dx.doi.org/10.1016/j.cult.2012.08.019
1556-858X/13/$ – see front matter

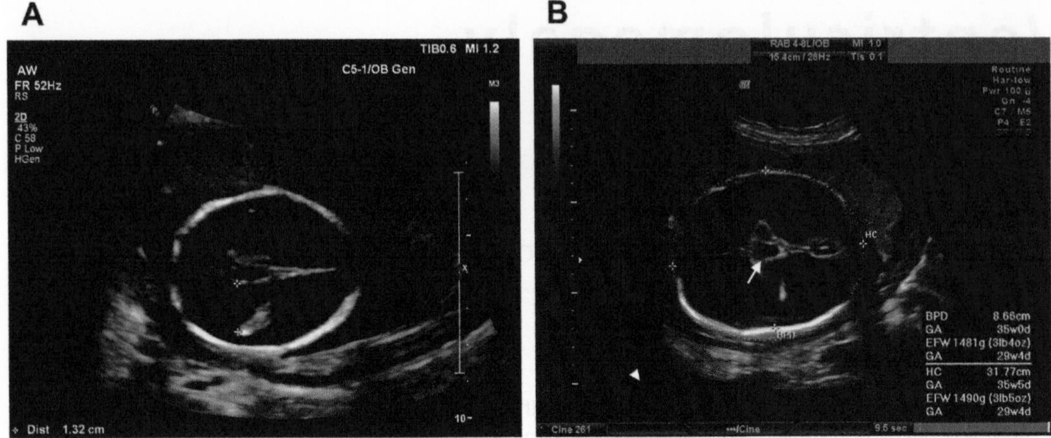

Fig. 1. Bilateral mild or moderate VM in an 18-week male fetus (*A*) and the same fetus in the third trimester (*B*). The third ventricle was noted to be dilated (*arrow*) with a normal fourth ventricle and cisterna magna. The patient opted for amniocentesis, which was positive for the L1CAM mutation, confirming a diagnosis of X-link aqueductal stenosis. After birth, the infant required ventriculo-peritoneal shunt placement.

restrict mild VM to diameters between 10 and 12 mm, which is also referred to as borderline VM (moderate 13–15 mm and severe >15 mm or ≥16 mm, **Box 1**). The terms ventriculomegaly and hydrocephalus can sometimes cause confusion. Hydrocephalus refers to a pathologic increase in cerebrospinal fluid volume (CSF), whereas VM is a generic term for ventricular enlargement due to a variety of causes. Since fetal ventricular pressure cannot be measured prenatally,[22] VM and hydrocephalus are frequently used to refer to lateral cerebral ventricular dilations between 10 and 15 mm and greater than 15 mm respectively.

WHAT ARE THE CAUSES OF CEREBRAL VM?

Every effort should be made to establish the etiology of VM, as the prognosis is quite variable. The list of causes is diverse and includes idiopathic causes, chromosomal disorders, genetic syndromes, viral infections, intraventricular hemorrhage, intracranial masses, obstruction, central nervous system malformations, and maldevelopment or destruction of cerebral tissue (**Table 1**). Regardless of the underlying cause, 1 of 3 processes explains the mechanism of ventricular enlargement: (1) increased relative fluid pressure within the ventricles in relation to the venous system because of decreased resorption or, rarely, increased production; (2) abnormal formation of fetal brain tissue resulting in an increase in ventricular size; or (3) atrophy of existing brain tissue.[22,23]

Box 1
Diagnostic criteria

Classification	Atrial Width
Mild or borderline	10–12 mm
Moderate	13–15 mm
Severe	>15 mm or ≥16 mm
or	
Mild	10–15 mm
Severe	>15 mm

The flow of CSF is predictable (**Fig. 2**). Blockage within the ventricular system, also known as noncommunicating hydrocephalus, can occur at any level but is most common at the aqueduct of Sylvius between the third and fourth ventricles. Careful evaluation of the ventricular system with attention to which parts of the system are normal and which are abnormal/dilated can help narrow down the cause, since the ventricular system distal to the point of obstruction will usually remain normal in appearance (**Fig. 2**). Aqueductal stenosis is suspected when the lateral and third ventricles are enlarged with a normal fourth ventricle. Correspondingly, obstruction on the foramina of Lushka and Magendie would appear as enlarged lateral, third, and fourth ventricles.[22]

Obstruction of the aqueduct of Sylvius can be caused by a number of genetic and other causes. X-linked aqueductal stenosis (Bickers-Adams syndrome), a form of congenital hydrocephalus, is a recessive condition caused by a mutation in the gene encoding L1 cell adhesion molecule (L1CAM) and characterized by aqueductal stenosis, mental retardation, paraperesis or paraplegia, and adducted thumbs. L1CAM mutations are also involved in the MASA spectrum (mental retardation, aphasia, shuffling gait, and adducted thumbs), X-linked spastic paraplegia type 1, and

Table 1
Causes of VM

Category	Disease	Cause of VM	Notes
Central nervous system anomalies	Congenital stenosis of the foramina of Monroe	a	Dilation of 1 or both lateral ventricles
	Spina bifida	a	Banana sign (obliteration of cisterna magna), lemon sign (scalloped frontal bones, open spinal defect, ↑AFP
	Dandy-Walker complex	a	Partial or complete absence of cerebellar vermis, dilated fourth ventricle, posterior fossa cyst
	Intracranial masses	a	Deforms parenchyma
	Arachnoid cyst	a	Extracerebral CSF-filled cyst
	Choroid plexus papilloma	b	Echogenic intraventricular mass with surface vascularity
	Vein of Galen aneurysm	b	
	Agenesis of the corpus callosum	c	Absent cavum septum pellucidum and pericallosal artery, teardrop shape of the lateral ventricle (colpocephaly)
	Holoprosencephaly	c	Incomplete division of the hemispheres
	Neuronal migration disorders	c	Lissencephaly (absent/reduced cerebral convolutions); schizencephaly (cortical mantle clefts)
	Neuronal proliferation disorders	c	Megalencephaly; microcephaly (head circumference >-2 to -3SD)
	Intracranial hemorrhage	a,d,e	Can be secondary to neonatal alloimmune thrombocytopenia
	Vascular insults	e	
	Sagittal sinus thrombosis	d	
	Porencephaly	e	
Aneuploidy	Trisomy 13,18,21	c	
Genetic syndromes	Congenital aqueductal stenosis	a	Dilation of both lateral ventricles and third ventricle, L1CAM (see **Fig. 1**)
	Apert syndrome		Craniosynostosis
	Miller-Dieker syndrome		Lissencephaly
	Seckel syndrome		Microcephalic osteodysplastic dwarfism
	Smith-Lemli-Opitz syndrome		Low estriol, disorder of cholesterol metabolism, microcephaly
	Walker-Warburg syndrome		Congenital muscular dystrophy, lissencephaly
	Neu-laxova syndrome		Agenesis of the corpus callosum
	Acrocallosal syndrome		Agenesis of the corpus callosum
	Aicardi syndrome		
Infections	CMV, toxoplasmosis Rubella Lymphocytic choriomeningitis visus *rarely*: mumps, enterovirus 71, parainfluenza virus type 3, parvovirus B19	a,d,e	Intracranial/periventricular echogenicities, Most common

Abbreviations: AFP, alpha fetoprotein; CMV, cytomegalovirus.
[a] Decreased CSF reabsorption, non-communicating.
[b] Increased CSF production.
[c] Abnormal formation of brain tissue.
[d] Decreased CSF reabsorption, communicating.
[e] Atrophy/destruction of existing brain tissue.
Adapted from Gaglioti P, Oberto M, Todros T. The significance of fetal ventriculomegaly: etiology, short- and long-term outcomes. Prenat Diagn 2009;29:33.

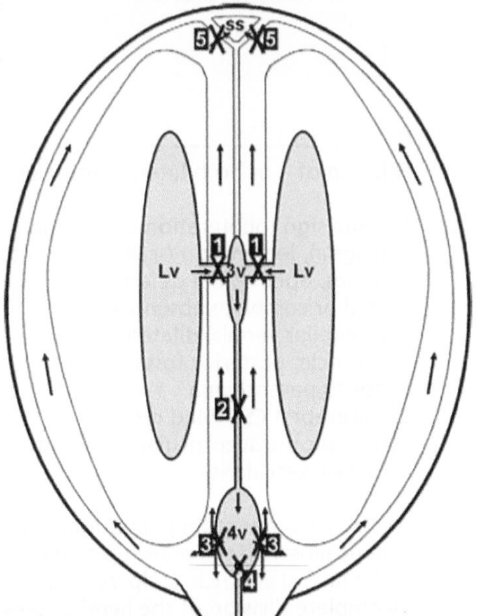

Fig. 2. CSF, produced by the choroid plexus, circulates in a predictable pathway, lateral ventricles → foramina of Monroe → third ventricle → aqueduct of Sylvius → fourth ventricle → spinal cord and subarachnoid spaces, before being reabsorbed into the ventricular system. Obstruction can occur at any point along this pathway, causing dilation proximal to the point of obstruction. (*From* Gaglioti P, Oberto M, Todros T. The significance of fetal ventriculomegaly: etiology, short- and long-term outcomes. Prenat Diagn 2009; 29:32; with permission.)

X-linked agenesis of the corpus callosum. If the family history suggests 1 of these disorders or the fetus is a male with isolated severe VM, DNA testing is warranted.[24]

Other causes of aqueductal stenosis include viral infection, intraventricular or intraparenchymal hemorrhage, masses, or malformations such as Chiari II. Viruses that have been most commonly linked to VM include cytomegalovirus, toxoplasmosis, and rubella, although several other viruses have been implicated (**Table 1**). Viral infection causes fibrosis of the aqueduct but can also prevent reabsorption of CSF at the arachnoid granulations (communicating hydrocephalus). Infections are found in 1% to 5% of cases of mild/moderate VM and 10% to 20% of cases of severe VM.[22,25] While other intracranial findings are often present, VM may be the only sign of infection. The preferred evaluation for infection is PCR of amniotic fluid; serology—although not as sensitive or specific—is a reasonable alternative if the patient declines amniocentesis or the amniocentesis was done previously and there is no sample available.[24]

Chromosomal anomalies such as trisomy 21 are another frequent cause of VM. Aneuploidy is responsible for more than 15% of cases of severe VM and 2.8% of cases of mild/moderate VM.[22,25] Trisomy 21 has a variable appearance on ultrasound; approximately half of fetuses will have no ultrasound findings, and in those that do, VM may be the only abnormality. For these reasons, amniocentesis for karyotype and chromosomal microarray analysis should be offered. The array of other causes of VM is shown in **Table 1**.

WHAT IS THE EMBRYOLOGY OF THE CEREBRAL VENTRICLES?

Development of the ventricular system begins with folding of the ectodermal neural plate to form the neural tube starting in the fourth embryonic week. The ventricular spaces are formed from the open cavity within the neural tube. During the sixth week, the telocele, the primitive neural cavity, within the telencephalon, or primitive forebrain, cleaves along the sagittal plane forming a pair of symmetric cavities.[26,27] Subsequent rotation and folding, and concomitant development of other intracranial structures, results in the definitive structure of the lateral ventricles.

WHAT IS THE ANATOMY OF THE CEREBRAL VENTRICLE?

The lateral ventricle is composed of the frontal horn (anterior), body, occipital horn (posterior), and temporal horn (inferior). The atrium of the lateral ventricle, also referred to as the trigone, is the portion where the body, occipital (posterior) horn, and temporal (inferior) horn converge.[16] The choroid plexus is formed from a fold in the medial wall of the lateral ventricle, which becomes covered with a pseudostratified epithelium. This epithelium ultimately forms the choroid plexus through further molding and proliferation of underlying blood vessel. The glomus of the choroid plexus is an enlargement of the choroid located within the atrium. CSF, produced by the choroid plexus, circulates from the lateral ventricles through foramina of Monroe into the third ventricle, and then through the cerebral aqueduct to the fourth ventricle. Fluid from the ventricular system then circulates into the spinal cord and subarachnoid spaces before being reabsorbed into the ventricular system.

BASIC 2-DIMENSIONAL IMAGING TECHNIQUE

The lateral ventricles can be clearly seen as early as 12 to 13 weeks; however, the atrial diameter is usually measured in the second trimester (typically starting at 16–18 weeks). In most cases, the lateral cerebral ventricles can be adequately visualized using transabdominal, 2D imaging. Several different methods of assessing the ventricle have been described. Measurement of the transverse diameter of the ventricular atrium in the transventricular view at the level of the glomus is currently favored (**Fig. 3**).[11,27]

Cardoza and colleagues[15] described a standardized method of measuring the ventricular diameter in 1988. They defined the plane of the transventricular view by the thalamus anteriorly and smooth posterior margin of the choroid plexus posteriorly. More recently, guidelines from the International Society of Obstetrics and Gynecology (ISUOG) defined the anterior landmarks as the cavum septum pellucidum and frontal (anterior) horns of the lateral ventricles.[11] Guibaud argued that the location of the glomus of the choroid plexus within the ventricle may change depending on the shape of the choroid plexus and suggested the fornix columns (base of the cavum septum pellucidum) anteriorly and the ambient cistern (cistern of the great cerebral veins) and internal parietal occipital sulcus posteriorly to improve measurement standardization.[28]

In addition to these landmarks, the midline structures should be perpendicular to the ultrasound beam, and the image should be sized such that the transventricular plane occupies the whole screen and both the proximal and distal calvarium are included. Typically in this plane, only the ventricle furthest from the transducer is clearly visualized due to artifact obscuring the more proximal hemisphere.[11,16] In a series of 608 consecutive ultrasounds, atrial measurements

Imaging protocol

- The lateral ventricles should be routinely assessed as part of the basic ultrasound
- Using 2-dimensional, gray-scale imaging, the lateral ventricle should be measured in the transventricular view
  - The transventricular view is defined by corpus callosum and frontal horns of the lateral ventricles anteriorly, and choroid plexus or ambient cistern posteriorly
  - The calvarium should occupy most of the screen
  - Midline structures should be equidistant from the calvarium and perpendicular to the ultrasound beam
- The diameter atrium should be measured perpendicular to the long access of the ventricle with the calipers placed at the inner edges of the ventricle wall
- The measurement is taken at the widest part of the atrium, but positioning the calipers at the parietal–occipital sulcus may improve reproducibility
- Measurements of atrial width in the coronal plane can be used when the atrium cannot be accurately measured in the transventricular view.
- The addition of 3-dimensional and Doppler images (based on physician/sonographer experience) may be of benefit in evaluating the anatomy of the central nervous system

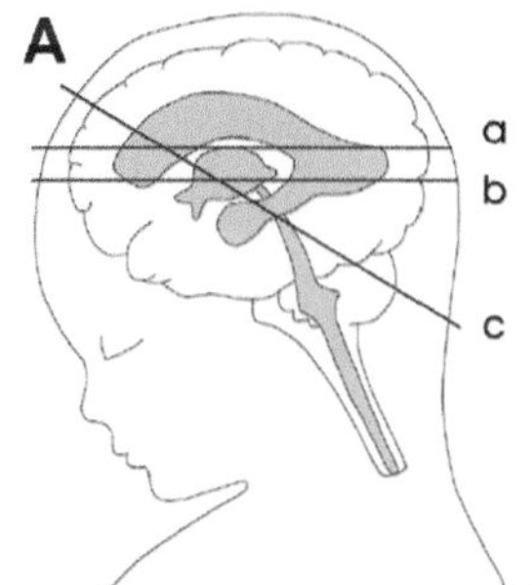

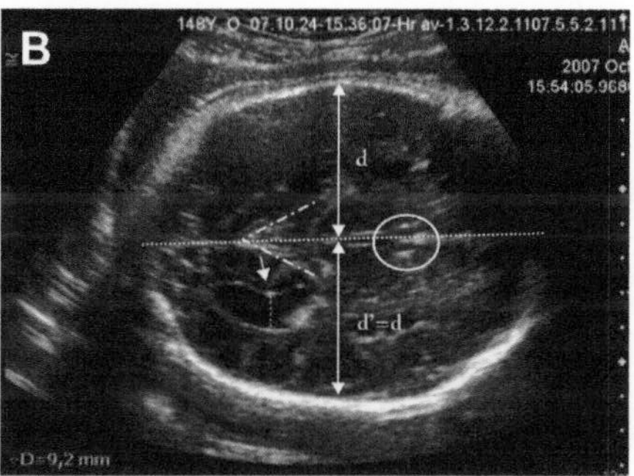

Fig. 3. The transventricular view. The diagram of the fetal head (*A*) shows the proper plane of the transventricular "a," transthalammic "b," and transcerebellar "c" views. The atrium of the lateral ventricles is measured an axial plane (*B*) through the frontal (anterior) horns and cavum septum pellucidum (fornix columns, *circle*) anteriorly, and posterior (occipital) horns posteriorly (V-shaped ambient cistern, dotted line; parietal–occipital sulcus, *arrow*). Some experts suggest using a plane slightly cephalic to that shown. (*From* Bornstein E, Monteagud A, Timor-Tritsch IE. The utilization of 3D and 4D technology in fetal neurosonology. Ultrasound Clinics 2008;(3): 497; with permisson; and Guibaud L. Fetal cerebral ventricular measurement and ventriculomegaly: time for procedure standardization. Ultrasound Obstet Gynecol 2009;34:128; with permission.)

were obtained in the transventricular view in 88% of cases.[13] In certain instances, the use of a transvaginal transducer may become necessary to assess the lateral ventricles such as when visualization is limited by maternal habitus or when the fetal head is deep in the pelvis. Additionally, transvaginal imaging may facilitate acquisition of sagittal and coronal planes and the higher transducer frequency permits improved resolution of intracranial structures when the fetus is in a cephalic lie.

In the transventricular plane, the atrium is almost entirely filled by the choroid plexus, which is easily recognizable by its brightly echogenic appearance. Shrinkage or compression of the choroid plexus and decreased filling of the atrium by the choroid plexus are other signs that are suggestive of VM. Some fluid between the choroid and ventricle walls is normal.[16,29,30] Hilpert and colleagues[13] demonstrated that atrial filling by the choroid plexus is always greater than 50% and greater than 60% in 98% of fetuses. The position of the choroid is dependent on gravity and rests against the lateral ventricle wall when the fetal head is transverse. When the lateral ventricle dilates, the choroid no longer rests against the lateral ventricle wall and takes on a "dangling" appearance.[29]

The diameter of the ventricular atrium is obtained by placing the calipers at the inner borders of the echoes created by the medial and lateral walls of the ventricle (ie, the junction of the ventricle wall and ventricle lumen, **Fig. 4**) perpendicular to the long axis of the ventricle.[11,28] Incorporating the suggestions of Guibaud to standardize measurement would have the effect on caliper placement shown in **Fig. 5**. Caliper placement perpendicular to midline structures or on or outside the echogenic reflection of the wall of the ventricle may lead to overestimation and a higher false-positive rate.[17] The interobserver variability is 3 mm,[17,31] which may be problematic at atrial widths close to 10 mm; in a series of fetuses referred for suspected VM, there was disagreement by a group of experienced radiologists in 10% of ultrasound studies.[31] When the atrium cannot be accurately measured in the transventricular view, precise measurements can be obtained in the coronal plane.[11,13] In 98% of fetuses, axial and coronal measurements differed by less than 2 mm.[13] Whereas in the transventricular plane only 1 ventricle is assessed because artifact obscures the near ventricle, both ventricles can be measured in the coronal plane.[32]

WHAT IS THE ROLE OF 3-DIMENSIONAL IMAGING OF THE FETAL CENTRAL NERVOUS SYSTEM?

The fetal central nervous system can be evaluated with transabdominal 3-dimensional (3D) ultrasound in the majority of cases,[33,34] and the saved volumes can be used for offline analysis and to facilitate telemedicine endeavors.[35] Standardized techniques for acquiring volumes have been described.[33,35–38] As with standard 2-dimensional imaging, decreased transmission is the most significant limiting factor; however, equipment, expertise, fetal position, and fetal movement can also contribute to inability to obtain good-quality images. Some of the proposed advantages of 3D imaging over standard 2-dimensional (2D) imaging are, among other things, the ability to store volumes for later review, simultaneous evaluation of multiple planes, and the ability to obtain volumetric measurements and tomographic planes similar those obtained by computed tomography (CT) or magnetic resonance imaging (MRI). Manipulation of acquired 3D

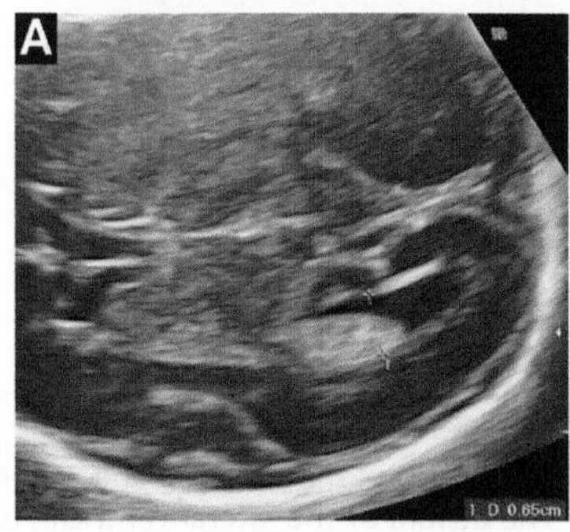

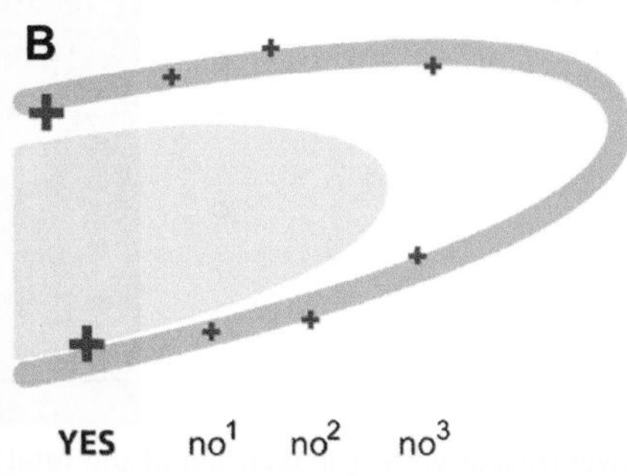

Fig. 4. (*A*) Measurement of atrium of the lateral ventricles. The calipers are positioned at the level of the glomus of the choroid plexus, inside the echoes generated by the ventricular walls. (*B*) Diagram to illustrate correct inner–inner placement of the calipers at the widest portion of the glomus of the choroid plexus. (*From* International Society of Ultrasound in Obstetrics and Gynecology Education Committee. Sonographic examination of the fetal central nervous system: guidelines for performing the 'basic examination' and the 'fetal neurosonogram'. Ultrasound Obstet Gynecol 2007;29:112; with permission.)

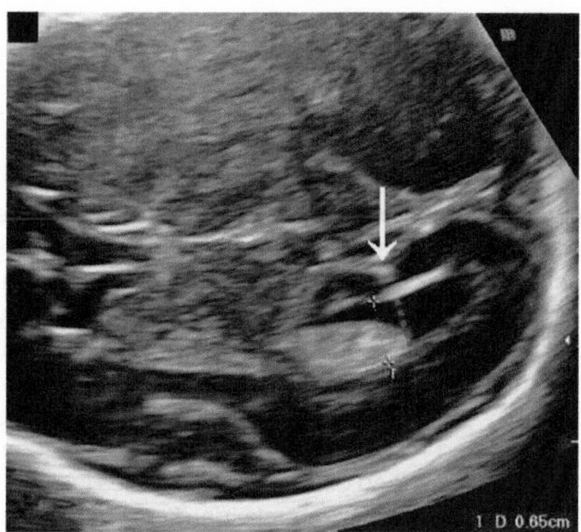

Fig. 5. Measurement of atrium of the lateral ventricles incorporating the International Society of Ultrasound in Obstetrics and Gynecology guidelines (ISUOG neurosonogram) and recommendations for caliper placement at the internal parieto-occipital sulcus proposed by Guibaud. (*From* International Society of Ultrasound in Obstetrics and Gynecology Education Committee. Sonographic examination of the fetal central nervous system: guidelines for performing the 'basic examination' and the 'fetal neurosonogram'. Ultrasound Obstet Gynecol 2007;29:112; with permission.)

volumes may facilitate evaluation of structures in the median sagittal plane such as the corpus callosum, which can be difficult to obtain with transabdominal 2D ultrasound.[38,39] However, there are limited data to support a distinct advantage of 3D ultrasound compared with standard 2D imaging. In a study of 11 fetuses with central nervous system anomalies, 3D imaging added to or changed the diagnosis in 2 (18%) cases.[40] Based on the available data, if the equipment and expertise are available, 3D ultrasound may be a useful supplement to 2D ultrasound when evaluating a fetus with VM.

WHAT IS THE RISK OF MORTALITY AND ADVERSE LONG-TERM NEURODEVELOPMENTAL OUTCOME?

Fetuses with VM are at risk of stillbirth, neonatal or infant death, and adverse long-term neurodevelopmental outcomes. It is generally agreed that survival decreases with increasing atrial width. Survival was inversely proportional to atrial width in a series of fetuses with VM; survival was 91%, 79%, and 75% when the atrial width was 10 to 12 mm, 12.1 to 14.9 mm, and greater than or equal to 15 mm, respectively.[41] Survival is also affected by the presence of other anomalies. For example, survival was 93% and 84% when the atrial width was 10 to 12 mm and greater than 12 mm, respectively but decreased to 60% when other anomalies were present.[42]

Neurodevelopmental outcome is more complicated. The outcome of fetuses with an identifiable cause (eg, spina bifida, Down syndrome) is defined by the specific etiology.[22] Nonetheless, the outcome of severe VM (atrial width ≥15mm) is typically poor. Breeze and colleagues[43] reported the outcomes of 20 cases of severe VM at presentation or progression to severe VM. Ten pregnancies were terminated and 10 were live born. Outcomes were evaluated at 4 months (and up to 2 years in most cases). Survival was 80% at 4 months. Of the survivors, 7 neonates were neurologically impaired (87.5%), and the 1 normally developing neonate was diagnosed with agenesis of the corpus callosum. Disabilities included abnormal vision, cerebral palsy, hemiparesis, seizures, and learning disability.

Associated cranial and extracranial anomalies are reportedly present in 58% to 65% of cases of severe VM,[40–42] with a greater than 15% risk of concomitant chromosomal anomalies when associated anomalies are found.[22] The likelihood of a normal neurologic outcome may improve when severe VM is isolated. In a report by Gaglioti and colleagues,[41] there were 13 terminations among 24 fetuses with isolated severe VM and 3 neonatal or infant deaths (72.7% survival). Of the 8 surviving neonates, neurologic development evaluated between ages 2 and 12 years was normal in 5 (62.5%). In contrast, normal neurologic outcomes were reported in only 11% to 12.5% of neonates (33%–40% developed mild neurologic morbidity) in 2 similar sized cohorts of neonates with isolated severe VM.[44,45]

The odds of normal long-term neurodevelopmental outcome have been reported to be between 81% and 100% when the atrial width is between 10 and 15 mm (pooled estimate 87%).[22,44,46–51] Several series have reported an association between the severity of VM and neurologic outcome.[41,47,48,52,53] For example, the neurologic outcome was normal in 93%, 75%, and 63% of surviving neonates with isolated mild (10–12 mm), moderate (12.1–14.9 mm), and severe (≥15 mm) VM present at birth.[41] Other series have reported similar rates of neurologic, motor, and cognitive impairment. Pooled estimates of the risk of abnormal long-term neurodevelopmental outcome are 4.9% to 7.7% for mild VM and 16.1% to 17.8% for moderate VM.[23,54,55] At least 1 study has challenged the appropriateness of a 10 mm cutoff. Signorelli and colleagues[56] studied 60 patients with isolated ventricular atrial diameters between

10 and 12 mm. In 38 cases, parents reported normal neurodevelopmental outcome between 3 and 10 years of age, and another 22 cases were found to be normal following formal evaluation at 12 and 18 months.

Regression, to either a lesser degree of VM or normal, has been noted in 38% to 47% of fetuses.[7,41] Beeghly and colleagues[42] performed a prospective study of patients with VM. Their methods included fetal MRI as part of the diagnostic protocol and formal neurodevelopmental testing at 6 months, 1 year, and 2 years. The authors found no association between the atrial width and risk of abnormal neurodevelopmental outcome including fetuses referred for VM seen on ultrasound in which the atria were normal on MRI, presumably due to measurement variability or regression. Their findings conflict with the notion that mild VM that regresses spontaneously is normal variant. Progression, on the other hand, is estimated to occur in 11% to 18% of cases and portends a worse outcome, including higher rates of chromosomal abnormalities and neurodevelopmental delay.[25,41,51] Lastly, a growing body of literature suggests that VM may be associated with subsequent development neuropsychiatric disorders including autism, attention-deficit hyperactivity disorder, learning disabilities, and schizophrenia. VM may be an early marker of abnormal cortical development; however, at present there is insufficient information to confirm this association.[24,25]

Caution should be used when offering counseling about the prognosis of apparently isolated VM. Postnatal evaluation will identify some cases of aneuploidy when a karyotype was not previously performed, and 10% to 13% of associated anomalies will not be recognized until after birth.[7,22,25] Comparison between studies is often limited by small, heterogeneous samples, varying definitions of VM, different inclusion criteria, different length of follow-up, and different methods used to assess neurodevelopmental outcome (which ranged from telephone interviews to formal neurologic testing). Among the features of VM, severe dilation (>15 mm), progression, and the presence of associated structural or chromosomal anomalies are most consistently associated with mortality and morbidity. In cases in which there is an identifiable cause, what is known about the underlying etiology will guide the counseling. In cases of apparently isolated VM, counseling is more difficult; there is no way to identify with certainty a fetus that will have a normal neurodevelopmental outcome or completely alleviate the anxiety connected to a diagnosis of VM.

SHOULD PATIENTS BE REFERRED FOR FETAL MRI?

Given the high incidence of associated abnormalities in fetuses with VM, fetal MRI has been suggested as an adjunct to ultrasound. Additionally, several outcome studies of isolated VM have included antenatal MRI in the evaluation. In nonselected fetuses with VM, MRI provided additional findings in 6% to 50% of cases.[57] In apparently isolated mild/moderate VM (10–15 mm), MRI provided additional information in 6% to 15% of cases[25,58–60] and in only 4% to 5% of fetuses with isolated mild VM (10–12 mm).[41,58] Additional diagnoses included cortical abnormalities (eg, heterotopias, hypoxic ischemia damage), abnormal gyration and sulcation, absence of the corpus callosum, absence of the cavum septum pellucidum, cerebellar abnormalities, mega cisterna magna, and open neural tube defects. On the other hand, MRI provided additional information in 10 of 12 cases (83%) of fetuses with VM and other central nervous system anomalies seen on ultrasound.[60]

The utility of MRI depends on many factors, including the severity of VM, gestational age, availability, and experience of sonographer/clinician. Referral bias probably accounts for some of the higher estimates. At least 1 study that included fetuses with mild-to-severe VM found additional anomalies in 50% of fetuses referred for MRI; however, only cases in which the ultrasound showed no additional anomalies but the clinician "instinctively felt there was a benefit to MRI" were referred.[61] MRI is more sensitive than ultrasound, especially when it comes to evaluation of neuronal migration and neuronal proliferation disorders, but cortical malformations are better evaluated at later gestational ages. This can be problematic when termination of pregnancy is being considered. MRI is probably not useful in cases that are known to be aneuploidy.

IS TREATMENT AVAILABLE?

At present, there is no role for in utero surgery. Manning and colleagues[62] reported 44 cases of ventriculo-amniotic shunts. The procedure-related death rate was 10%, and the perinatal mortality rate was 17%. Among survivors, 66% experienced moderate-to-severe handicaps. Their results did not represent an improvement over expectant management, which led to a de facto moratorium on the procedure. Although the use of cephalocentesis to drain the ventricles and prevent compression of the cortex has been reported, the current role of

Pearls, pitfalls, and variants

	Description	Reference
Pearls		
Evaluation of the ventricular system	Circulation of CSF is predictable; evaluation of the ventricular system noting the normal and abnormal/dilated parts may narrow down the possible etiologies	22
Dangling choroid	The choroid plexus is attached at the foramen of Monro and rests on the dependent ventricle wall. The choroid angle, the angle of the long axis of the choroid relative to the midline, is increased in VM giving the choroid a "dangling" appearance; larger angles indicate greater degrees of VM	29
Identification of the ventricle wall	The lateral wall of the ventricle may be obscured by the more echogenic choroid plexus. In all but the most severe cases of VM, the choroid in the dependent ventricle will rest against the lateral wall, aiding in identification	29
Error overestimate atrial width	Errors in ascertainment of the ventricular size are less likely to be an underestimate	17
Standards for measurement	Use of standardized criteria for image ascertainment and atrial measurement may reduce error and increase reproducibility	11,13,28
Pitfalls		
Misidentification of the ventricle walls	Anechoic brain tissue surrounding the ventricle can be misinterpreted as CSF The pia-arachnoid at the base of the lateral fissure generates a reflection that can be mistaken for the wall of the lateral ventricle, leading to misdiagnosis of VM **(Fig. 6)**	29
Improper plane selection	An off-axis image will overestimate the ventricle size, leading to false-positive results	17
Improper caliper placement	Placement of the calipers too posteriorly can lead to overestimation of ventricle size due to focal dilation of the occipital horn in the third trimester	28
Interobserver variability	The interobserver variability is 3 mm among experienced obstetric radiologists, which may lead to disagreement when atrial widths are close to 10 mm	31
Variants		
Large choroid plexus cysts	Isolated, large choroid plexus cysts that dilate the ventricle, giving the appearance of VM, are unlikely to be clinically significant	24
Effect of gender	Atrial diameter is slightly but significantly larger in males; despite the difference, gender lacks prognostic significance	14,18,63,64
Asymmetry	A small amount of ventricular asymmetry is normal	2,63
Unilateral VM	Visualization of only 1 ventricle in the transventricular view may miss cases of unilateral VM.	

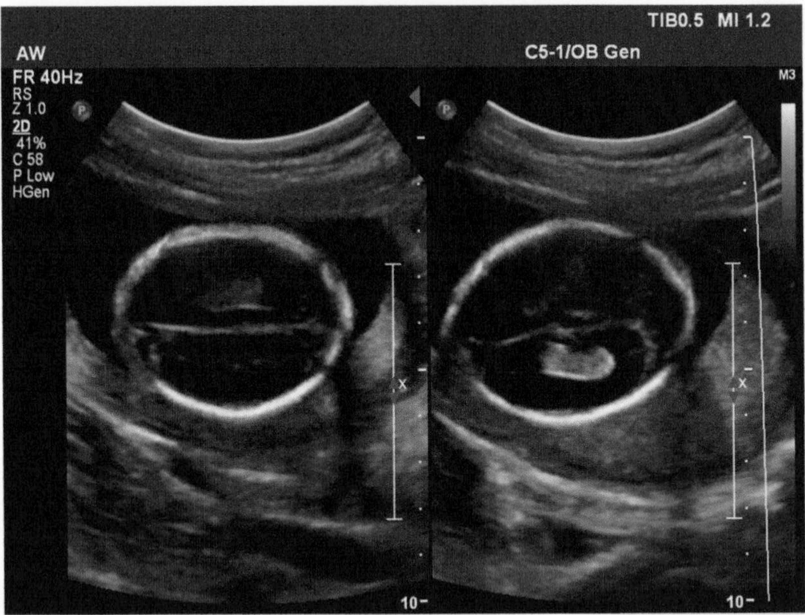

Fig. 6. The axial view on the right demonstrates how normal, anechoic brain tissue could be mistaken for VM. When the falx is perpendicular to the ultrasound, the choroid will rest against the lateral ventricle wall. In this image, the normal angle of the choroid suggests that the ventricle is normal.

cephalocentesis is as a destructive procedure done to prevent maternal morbidity by permitting vaginal delivery.

SUMMARY

The diagnosis of fetal cerebral VM is made when the diameter of the fetal cerebral ventricles are at least 10 mm. Central nervous system anomalies can elicit emotions unlike any other anomalies, and even if the diagnosis is not confirmed, it may be impossible to completely relieve parents' anxiety. A thorough knowledge of the recommended imaging guidelines and sources of measurement error is essential. Given the frequent association with other anomalies and diverse group of causes, a detailed evaluation is required. MRI is controversial, due to the high cost and potentially low yield; however, an MRI may be justifiable in certain cases such as severe VM or when associated central nervous system anomalies cannot be excluded by a detailed

What the referring physician needs to know

For suspected fetal cerebral VM, the referring physician should:

Complete a basic fetal ultrasound and detailed anatomic ultrasound with special attention to the intracranial structures and spine

Obtain a brief history (eg, family history, recent illness)

Obtain results of aneuploidy screening or, if not done, discuss screening

Arrange for a repeat evaluation to reassess ventricular size and detect anomalies that may have been missed previously; the optimal timing and frequency of follow-up is not well studied

There are no data to support the use of fetal monitoring (eg, nonstress tests) for VM in the absence of other indications

Cesarean section should be reserved for the usual indications except when the fetal head circumference is enlarged; cesarean section should be considered with an absolute head circumference of 40 cm or more

Cephalocentesis to decompress the head can be offered to women who wish to avoid the risks of cesarean section, but this often results in fetal death[65]

ultrasound. Despite careful evaluation, a number of neonates will be found to have been incompletely diagnosed after birth. VM increases the risk of stillbirth and neonatal/infant death, and survivors are at risk for long-term neurodevelopmental abnormalities.

REFERENCES

1. Filly RA, Goldstein RB, Callen PW. Fetal ventricle: importance in routine obstetric sonography. Radiology 1991;181:1–7.
2. Achiron R, Schimmel M, Achiron A, et al. Fetal mild idiopathic ventriculomegaly: is there a correlation with fetal trisomy? Ultrasound Obstet Gynecol 1993;84:110–4.
3. Alagappan R, Browing PD, Laorr A, et al. Distal lateral ventricular atrium: revaluation of normal range. Radiology 1994;193:405–8.
4. Kinzler WL, Smulian JC, McLean DA, et al. Outcome of prenatally diagnosed mild unilateral cerebral ventriculomegaly. J Ultrasound Med 2001;20:257–62.
5. Mailath-Pokorny M, Tauscher V, Krampl-Bettelheim E, et al. Fetal cerebral ventriculomegaly: prenatal diagnosis, chromosomal abnormalities and associated anomalies in 146 fetuses. Ultrasound Obstet Gynecol 2009;34(Suppl 1):177–284.
6. Myrianthopoulos NC. Epidemiology of central nervous system malformations. In: Vinken PJ, Bruyn GW, editors. Handbook of clinical neurology. Amsterdam (The Netherlands): Elsevier; 1977. p. 139–71.
7. Sethna F, Tennant PW, Rankin J, et al. Prevalence, natural history, and clinical outcome of mild to moderate ventriculomegaly. Obstet Gynecol 2001; 117:867–76.
8. McGahan JP, Phillips HE. Ultrasonic evaluation of the size of the trigone of the fetal ventricle. J Ultrasound Med 1983;2:315–9.
9. American College of Obstetricians and Gynecologists (ACOG). Ultrasonography in pregnancy. ACOG technical bulletin 187. Washington, DC: ACOG; 1993.
10. American Institute of Ultrasound in Medicine. AIUM practice guideline for the performance of obstetric ultrasound examinations. J Ultrasound Med 2010; 29:157–66.
11. International Society of Ultrasound in Obstetrics and Gynecology Education Committee. Sonographic examination of the fetal central nervous system: guidelines for performing the 'basic examination' and the 'fetal neurosonogram'. Ultrasound Obstet Gynecol 2007;29:109–16.
12. Almog B, Gamzu R, Achiron R, et al. Fetal lateral ventricular width: what should be its upper limit? A prospective cohort study and reanalysis of the current and previous data. J Ultrasound Med 2003; 22:39–43.
13. Hilpert PL, Hall BE, Kurtz AB. The atria of the fetal lateral ventricles: a sonographic study of normal atrial size and choroid plexus volume. AJR Am J Roentgenol 1995;163:731–4.
14. Salomon LJ, Bernard JP, Ville Y. Reference ranges for fetal ventricular width: a non-normal approach. Ultrasound Obstet Gynecol 2007;30:61–6.
15. Cardoza JD, Goldstein RB, Filly RA. Exclusion of fetal ventriculomegaly with a single measurement: the width of the lateral ventricular atrium. Radiology 1988;3:85–7.
16. Pilu GL, Reece EA, Goldstein I, et al. Sonographic evaluation of the normal developmental anatomy of fetal cerebral ventricles: II. The atria. Obstet Gynecol 1989;73:250–6.
17. Heiserman J, Filly RA, Goldstein RB. Effect of measurement errors on the sonographic evaluation of ventriculomegaly. J Ultrasound Med 1991;10:121–4.
18. Patel MD, Goldstein RB, Tung S, et al. Fetal cerebral ventricular atrium: difference in size according to sex. Radiology 1995;194:713–5.
19. Farrell TA, Hertzberg BS, Kliewer MA, et al. Lateral ventricles: reassessment of normal values for atrial diameter at US. Radiology 1994;193:409–11.
20. Siedler DE, Filly RA. Relative growth of the higher fetal brain structures. J Ultrasound Med 1987;6:573–6.
21. Snijders RJ, Nicolaides KH. Fetal biometry at 14–40 weeks' gestation. Ultrasound Obstet Gynecol 1994; 4:34–48.
22. Gaglioti P, Oberto M, Todros T. The significance of fetal ventriculomegaly: etiology, short- and long-term outcomes. Prenat Diagn 2009;29:381–8.
23. Bronsteen RA, Comstock CH. Central nervous system anomalies. Clin Perinatol 2000;27:791–812.
24. Norton M. Fetal ventriculomegaly. In: Basow DS, editor. UpToDate. Waltham (MA): UpToDate; 2012.
25. Melchiorre K, Bhide A, Gika AD, et al. Counseling in mild ventriculomegaly. Ultrasound Obstet Gynecol 2009;34:212–24.
26. Goldstein I, Reece EA, Pilu GL, et al. Sonographic evaluation of the normal developmental anatomy of fetal cerebral ventricles: I. The frontal horn. Obstet Gynecol 1988;72:588–92.
27. Pilu G, Perolo A, Falco P, et al. Ultrasound of the fetal central nervous system. Curr Opin Obstet Gynecol 2000;12:93–103.
28. Guibaud L. Fetal cerebral ventricular measurement and ventriculomegaly: time for procedure standardization. Ultrasound Obstet Gynecol 2009;34:127–30.
29. Cardoza JD, Filly RA, Podransky AE. The dangling choroid plexus: a sonographic observation of value in excluding ventriculomegaly. AJR Am J Roentgenol 1988;151:767–70.
30. Mahony BS, Nyberg DA, Hirsch JH, et al. Mild idiopathic lateral cerebral ventricular dilatation in utero: sonographic evaluation. Radiology 1988;169: 715–21.

31. Levine D, Feldman HA, Tannus JF, et al. Frequency and cause of disagreements in diagnoses for fetuses referred for ventriculomegaly. Radiology 2008;247:516–27.
32. Garel C, Alberti C. Coronal measurement of the fetal ventricles: comparison between ultrasonography and magnetic resonance imaging. Ultrasound Obstet Gynecol 2006;27:23–7.
33. Correa FF, Lara C, Bellver J, et al. Examination of the fetal brain by transabdominal three-dimensional ultrasound: potential for routine neurosonographic studies. Ultrasound Obstet Gynecol 2006;27:503–8.
34. Endres LK, Cohen L. Reliability and validity of three-dimensional fetal brain volumes. J Ultrasound Med 2001;20:1265–9.
35. Bornstein E, Monteagudo A, Santos R, et al. Basic as well as detailed neurosonograms can be performed by offline analysis of three-dimensional fetal brain volumes. Ultrasound Obstet Gynecol 2010;36:20–5.
36. Viñals F, Muñoz M, Naveas R, et al. Transfrontal three-dimensional visualization of midline cerebral structures. Ultrasound Obstet Gynecol 2007;30:162–8.
37. Timor-Tritsch IE, Monteagudo A, Mayberry P. Three-dimensional ultrasound evaluation of the fetal brain: the three horn view. Ultrasound Obstet Gynecol 2000;16:302–6.
38. Pilu G, Segata M, Ghi T, et al. Diagnosis of midline anomalies of the fetal brain with the three-dimensional median view. Ultrasound Obstet Gynecol 2006;27:522–9.
39. Wang PH, Ying TH, Wang PC, et al. Obstetrical three-dimensional ultrasound in the visualization of the intracranial midline and corpus callosum of fetuses with cephalic position. Prenat Diagn 2000;20:518–20.
40. Mueller GM, Weiner CP, Yankowitz J. Three-dimensional ultrasound in the valuation of fetal head and spine anomalies. Obstet Gynecol 1996;88:372–8.
41. Gaglioti P, Danelon D, Bontempo S, et al. Fetal cerebral ventriculomegaly: outcome in 176 cases. Ultrasound Obstet Gynecol 2005;25:372–7.
42. Beeghly M, Ware J, Soul J, et al. Neurodevelopmental outcome of fetuses referred for ventriculomegaly. Ultrasound Obstet Gynecol 2010;35:405–16.
43. Breeze AC, Alexander PM, Murdoch EM, et al. Obstetric and neonatal outcomes in severe fetal ventriculomegaly. Prenat Diagn 2007;27:124–9.
44. Graham E, Duhl A, Ural S, et al. The degree of antenatal ventriculomegaly is related to pediatric neurological morbidity. J Matern Fetal Med 2001;10:258–63.
45. Kennelly MM, Cooley SM, McParland PJ. Natural history of apparently isolated severe fetal ventriculomegaly: perinatal survival and neurodevelopmental outcome. Prenat Diagn 2009;29:1135–40.
46. Patel MD, Filly AL, Hersh DR, et al. Isolated mild fetal cerebral ventriculomegaly: clinical course and outcome. Radiology 1994;192:759–64.
47. Bloom SL, Bloom D, Dellanebbia C, et al. The developmental outcome of children with antenatal mild isolated ventriculomegaly. Obstet Gynecol 1997;90:93–7.
48. Vergani P, Locatelli A, Strobelt N, et al. Clinical outcome of mild fetal ventriculomegaly. Am J Obstet Gynecol 1998;178:218–22.
49. Pilu G, Falco P, Gabrielli S, et al. The clinical significance of fetal isolated cerebral borderline ventriculomegaly: report of 31 cases and review of the literature. Ultrasound Obstet Gynecol 1999;14:320–6.
50. Breeze AC, Dey PK, Lees CC, et al. Obstetric and neonatal outcomes in apparently isolated mild fetal ventriculomegaly. J Perinat Med 2005;33(3):236–40.
51. Ouahba J, Luton D, Vuillard E, et al. Prenatal isolated mild ventriculomegaly: outcome in 167 cases. BJOG 2006;113:1072–9.
52. Falip C, Blanc N, Maes E, et al. Prenatal clinical and imaging follow-up of infants with prenatal isolated mild ventriculomegaly: a series of 101 cases. Pediatr Radiol 2007;37:981–9.
53. Laskin MD, Kingdom J, Toi A, et al. Perinatal and neurodevelopmental outcome with isolated fetal ventriculomegaly: a systematic review. J Matern Fetal Neonatal Med 2005;18:289.
54. Chan LW, Lau TK. Re: counseling in isolated mild fetal ventriculomegaly. Ultrasound Obstet Gynecol 2010;35:624–5.
55. [Erratum]. Ultrasound Obstet Gynecol 2010;35:626.
56. Signorelli M, Tiberti A, Valseriati D, et al. Width of the fetal lateral ventricular atrium between 10 and 12 mm: a simple variation of the norm? Ultrasound Obstet Gynecol 2004;23:14–8.
57. Griffiths PD, Reeves MJ, Morris JE, et al. A prospective study of fetuses with isolated ventriculomegaly investigated by antenatal sonography and in utero MR imaging. AJNR Am J Neuroradiol 2010;31:106–11.
58. Salomon LJ, Ouahba J, Delezoide AL, et al. Third-trimester fetal MRI in isolated 10- to 12-mm ventriculomegaly: is it worth it? BJOG 2006;113:942–7.
59. Valsky DV, Ben-Sira L, Porat S, et al. The role of magnetic resonance imaging in the evaluation of isolated mild ventriculomegaly. J Ultrasound Med 2004;23:519–23.
60. Benacerraf BR, Shipp TD, Bromley B, et al. What does magnetic resonance imaging add to the prenatal sonographic diagnosis of ventriculomegaly? J Ultrasound Med 2007;26:1513–22.
61. Morris JE, Rickard S, Paley MN, et al. The value of in-utero magnetic resonance imaging in ultrasound diagnosed foetal isolated cerebral venticulomegaly. Clin Radiol 2007;62:140–4.
62. Manning FA, Harrison MR, Rodeck C. Catheter shunts for fetal hydronephrosis and hydrocephalus.

Report of the international fetal surgery registry. N Engl J Med 1986;315:336–40.

63. Kivilevitch Z, Achiron R, Zalel Y. Fetal brain asymmetry: in utero sonographic study of normal fetuses. Am J Obstet Gynecol 2010;202: 359.e1–8.

64. Nadel AS, Benacerraf BR. Lateral ventricular atrium: larger in male than female fetuses. Int J Gynaecol Obstet 1995;51:123–6.

65. Chasen ST, Chervenak F, McCullough LB. The role of cephalocentesis in modern obstetrics. Am J Obstet Gynecol 2001;185:734–6.

Ultrasonography for Cesarean Scar Ectopics

Dzhamala Gilmandyar, MD

KEYWORDS

- Cesarean scar ectopics • Abnormal pregnancy implantation • Extrauterine gestation
- Transvaginal ultrasonography

KEY POINTS

- Cesarean scar ectopic pregnancy is a rare form of abnormal pregnancy implantation.
- Accurate early diagnosis is vital to decrease maternal morbidity.
- Transvaginal ultrasonography is an essential tool in diagnosis.
- Diagnostic imaging criteria can be very helpful in distinguishing this from other forms of anomalous gestations.

OVERVIEW AND CLINICAL SIGNIFICANCE

Cesarean scar ectopic (CSE) is an extrauterine gestation implanted within the previous surgical site and surrounded by myometrial tissue. Although the incidence is thought to have increased over the last 10 years, it is still a fairly rare occurrence. For this reason, much of the data that currently exists is in the form of case reports. A recent report reviewed 59 articles that collectively included 112 cases.[1] The estimated incidence was found to be 1:1800 to 1:2216 over the last 10 years, and the frequency of occurrence did not appear to be related to the number of prior cesarean deliveries or the time elapsed since the surgery.[2] More than 50% of CSE cases had only 1 previous cesarean, and the time from last cesarean and current CSE ranged between 6 months and 12 years.[1,3] Prior cesarean is a major risk factor, although any uterine surgery or manipulation, such as myomectomy or dilation and curettage, can predispose a woman to CSE.[2]

Although the exact cause remains unknown, theories exist about the possible etiology of this pathologic gestation. The most prevalent theory is that embryonic tissue migrates through a microscopic tract within the scar tissue and adheres to an extrauterine location while remaining surrounded by the myometrium.[2]

Early diagnosis is essential because an unrecognized and untreated CSE can be a life-threatening condition. Fortunately most are found in the first trimester, between 5 and 12 weeks, and treatment is initiated before rupture in the majority of cases.[3] Although more than one-third of these pregnancies are asymptomatic, the most common presentation is painless vaginal bleeding (38.6%), followed by abdominal pain with bleeding (15.8%) and abdominal pain without bleeding (8.8%).[1]

DIAGNOSTIC CRITERIA

Diagnosis can be challenging, but transvaginal ultrasonography has proved to be extremely beneficial, with an estimated sensitivity rate of 84.6%.[1] Some investigators have suggested using a combined approach of transvaginal and transabdominal imaging for more optimal visualization and a "panoramic" view.[4] A practical approach is

Disclosures: The author has no conflicts of interest.
Department of Obstetrics and Gynecology, University of Rochester School of Medicine, 601 Elmwood Avenue, Box 668, Rochester, NY 14642, USA
E-mail address: dzhamala_gilmandyar@urmc.rochester.edu

Ultrasound Clin 8 (2013) 27–30
http://dx.doi.org/10.1016/j.cult.2012.08.011
1556-858X/13/$ – see front matter

to perform transvaginal ultrasonography for a detailed evaluation, followed by a transabdominal scan with a filled bladder to help delineate the interface between the CSE and bladder.

Several experts have concurred on specific sonographic diagnostic criteria for CSE, which help in distinguishing it from other forms of abnormal pregnancies[3–6]:

1. Absence of intrauterine tissue with visible and empty endometrial cavity (**Fig. 1**)
2. Absence of embryonic tissue within the endocervical canal (**Figs. 2** and **3**)
3. Presence of gestational sac (with or without fetus and cardiac activity) within the anterior isthmic part of the uterus (**Figs. 4** and **5**)
4. Absence or reduction in thickness of the myometrium between the bladder and the gestational sac (see **Fig. 4**; **Fig. 6**)

IMAGING FINDINGS

Myometrium Between the Bladder and Gestational Sac

In most cases, the myometrial thickness between the bladder and the gestational sac is less than 5 mm[7] (this can be seen in **Fig. 6**). Some reports have found a bulging of the sac through an actual defect in the myometrium.[8]

Doppler Studies

Jurkovic and colleagues[9,10] suggested adding Doppler studies to help differentiate between viable and nonviable pregnancies, because this would affect further management. It is also helpful in determining the relationship of the pregnancy to bladder, a more precise location within the scar, and the degree of vascularity and blood flow within the pregnancy. **Fig. 7** shows a Doppler study of the patient seen in **Figs. 5** and **6**. The prominent vasculature surrounding the gestation as well as cardiac flow can be seen. On Doppler interrogation, one can usually appreciate a high-velocity (peak systolic velocity >20 cm/s) and low impedance (pulsatility index <1) flow.[10]

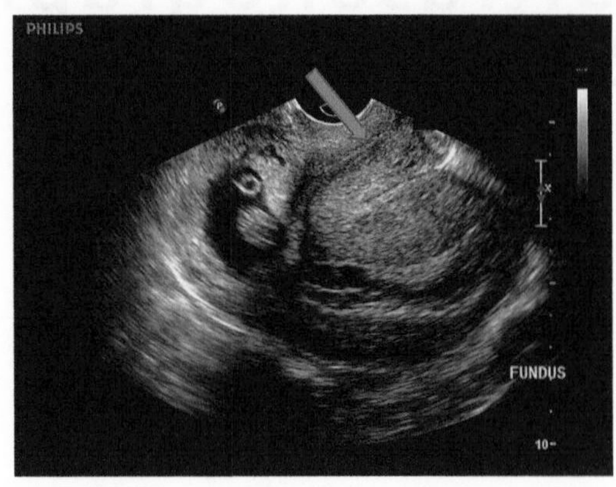

Fig. 2. Empty cervical canal (*blue arrow*).

Three-Dimensional Ultrasonography

Three-dimensional (3D) ultrasonography is a more recent tool used in evaluating pregnancies. Because CSE is a rare event, few reports exist on use of 3D sonography in assessing this particular type of pregnancy. From the published data, 3D sonography in CSE assessment does not appear to be essential in establishing the diagnosis, but can be helpful in recognizing subtle anatomic details.[11] Enhanced visualization of the myometrial thickness and distance from the bladder, as well as the shape of gestational sac, are advantages of 3D imaging.[11] Chou and colleagues[12] suggested its use and superiority in comparison with conventional 2D imaging, in evaluating resolution of the

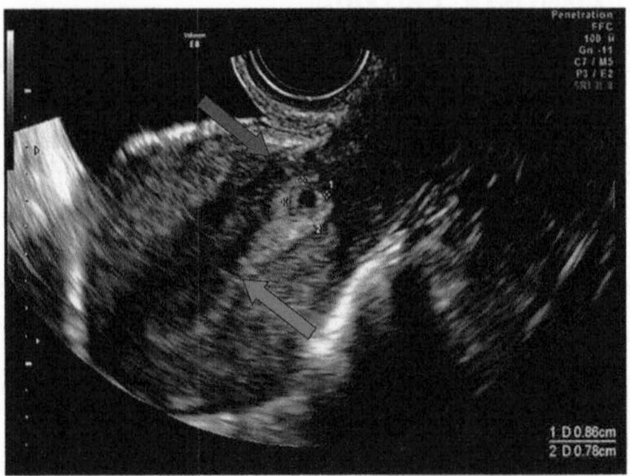

Fig. 1. Sagittal view illustrating a gestational sac in the anterior isthmic part of the uterus. Note the empty endometrium (*green arrow*) and a thin myometrium between the sac and the bladder (*blue arrow*).

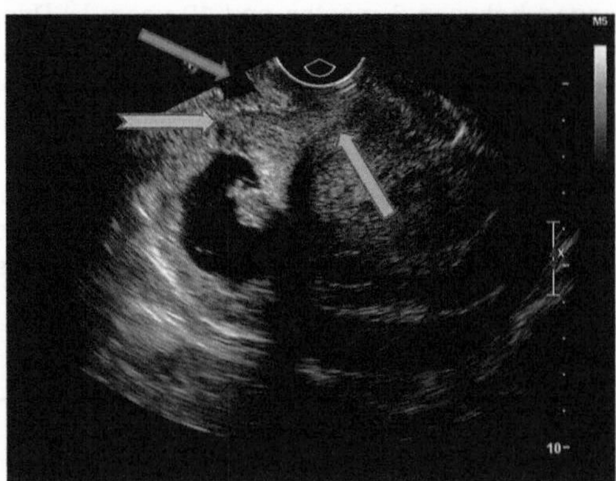

Fig. 3. Empty cervical canal (*green arrow*) in relationship to the gestation and the surrounding thin myometrium (*yellow arrow*) and bladder (*blue arrow*).

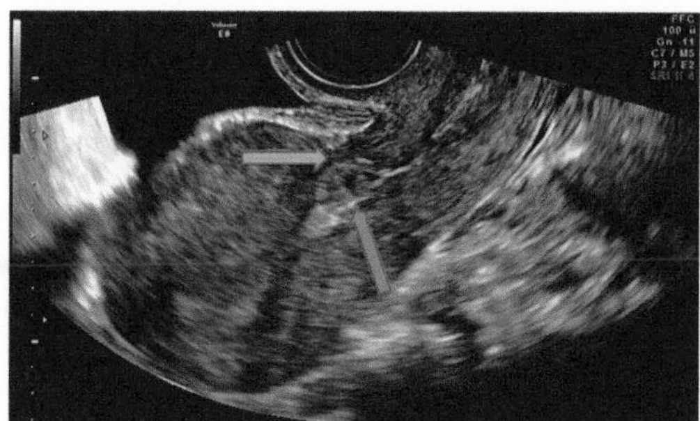

Fig. 4. Gestational sac within the anterior isthmic portion of the uterus (*blue arrow*) and the thin myometrium separating it from the bladder (*green arrow*).

ectopic after treatment, and reported improved visualization of the gestational-sac volume.

Sliding Organ Sign

Jurkovic and colleagues[9] recommended using the "sliding organ sign" in assisting with the diagnosis of CSE. This term refers to lack of movement of the gestational sac with pressure applied by the transabdominal probe. Other investigators have discouraged this practice because of the fear of incidental rupture or disruption of vasculature, and subsequent bleeding.

COMMON PITFALLS AND VARIANTS

Several types of anomalous gestations can be mistaken for CSE. In general, following the aforementioned guidelines and diagnostic criteria should help avoid some of the pitfalls, but these diagnoses should still be kept in mind when evaluating for CSE.

Cervical Pregnancy

Cervicoisthmic pregnancy is even rarer than CSE, with an incidence of about 1 in 9000.[13] While it is usually possible to visualize some gestational tissue within the canal and a ballooned cervical canal, the main differentiation from CSE is a typically intact layer of myometrium between the bladder and gestational sac. **Fig. 8** illustrates these findings.[14]

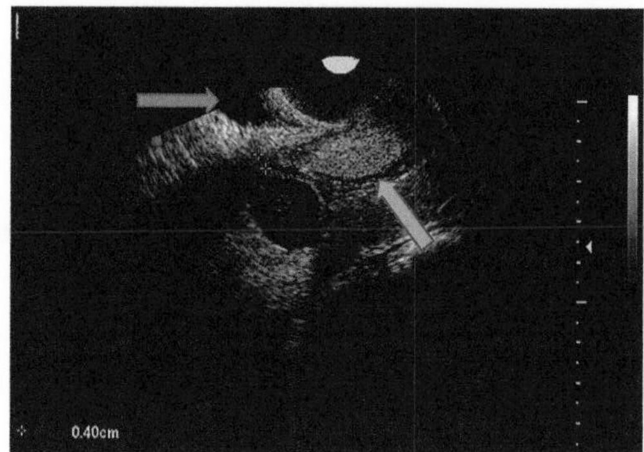

Fig. 6. Thin myometrium measuring 4 mm (*calipers*) separating the gestational sac from the bladder (*blue arrow*). Note the empty cervical canal (*green arrow*).

Spontaneous Miscarriage

Doppler interrogation becomes very useful in differentiating a miscarriage in progress from CSE. Because the location of a gestational sac in the process of being expelled from the uterus can vary at the time of the ultrasound scan, lack of vascular flow is key in differentiating it from CSE, which is well perfused.

Placenta Accreta

Placenta accreta refers to abnormal placental implantation of various degrees within the myometrium. Placenta accreta is visualized as being due to defective or absent decidua, and is thought to have some relation to anatomic defect of previous

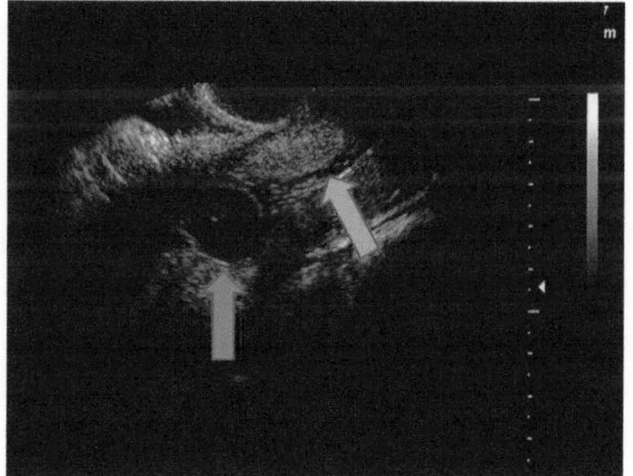

Fig. 5. Gestational sac with a yolk sac and fetal pole (*blue arrow*) in the anterior isthmic portion of the uterus, and an empty cervical canal (*green arrow*).

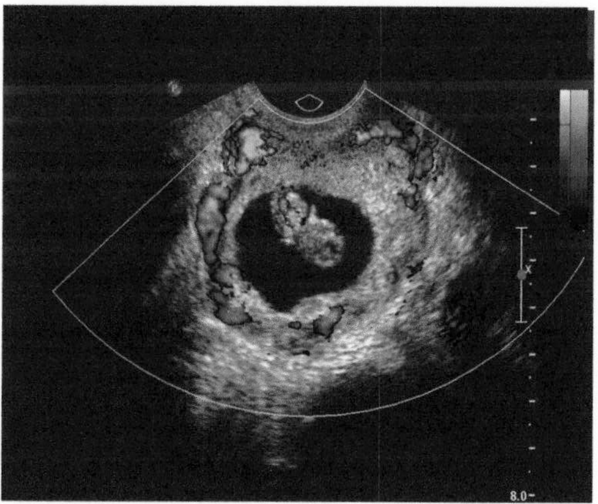

Fig. 7. Doppler study of the patient seen in **Figs. 5** and **6**. Note the vascular flow and cardiac activity.

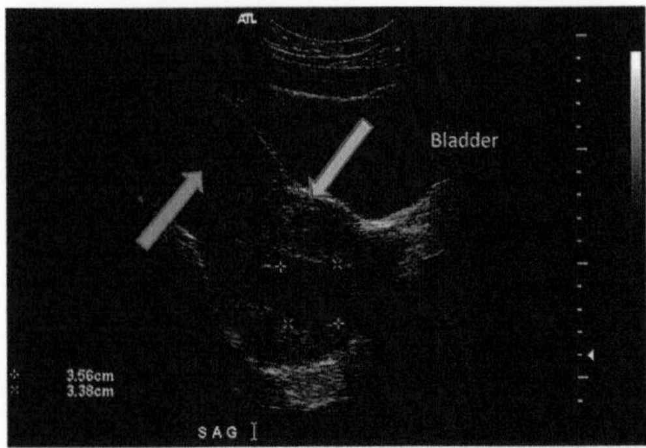

Fig. 8. Sagittal view of the uterus and cervix. Note the gestational sac in the ballooning cervical canal (*calipers*), empty uterus (*blue arrow*), and intact myometrium (*green arrow*).

scar and abnormal migration of trophoblastic tissue through that tract, similar to CSE. The important differentiation between this entity and CSE is that in the case of placenta accreta, the actual pregnancy is intrauterine and can be visualized within the endometrial cavity.

SUMMARY

Although CSE affects only a small number of women, its undiagnosed presence can be hazardous to maternal health. Early detection is crucial for improving prognosis and decreasing maternal morbidity. In general, CSE has specific sonographic features that allow for accurate early diagnosis with transvaginal ultrasonography. Use of transvaginal ultrasonography has led to most CSE pregnancies being identified in the first trimester, followed by timely intervention and ultimate optimization of outcomes.

REFERENCES

1. Rotas MA, Haberman S, Levgur M. Cesarean scar ectopic pregnancies: etiology, diagnosis, and management. Obstet Gynecol 2006;107:1373.
2. Ash A, Smith A, Maxwell D. Caesarean scar pregnancy. BJOG 2007;114:253.
3. Seow KM, Huang LW, Lin YH, et al. Caesarean scar pregnancy: issues in management. Ultrasound Obstet Gynecol 2004;23:247–53.
4. Maymon R, Halperin R, Mendlovic S, et al. Ectopic pregnancies in a caesarean scar: review of the medical approach to an iatrogenic complication. Hum Reprod Update 2004;10:515–23.
5. Godin PA, Bassil S, Donnez J. An ectopic pregnancy developing in a previous caesarian section scar. Fertil Steril 1997;67:398–400.
6. Fylstra DL. Ectopic pregnancy within a cesarean scar: a review. Obstet Gynecol Surv 2002;57:537–43.
7. Weimin W, Wenqing L. Effect of early pregnancy on a previous lower segment cesarean section scar. Int J Gynaecol Obstet 2002;77:201–7.
8. Einenkel J, Stumpp P, Ko S, et al. A misdiagnosed case of caesarean scar pregnancy. Arch Gynecol Obstet 2005;271:178–81.
9. Jurkovic D, Hillaby K, Woelfer B, et al. First-trimester diagnosis and management of pregnancies implanted into the lower uterine segment cesarean section scar. Ultrasound Obstet Gynecol 2003;21: 220–7.
10. Jurkovic D, Jauniaux E, Kurjak A, et al. Transvaginal color Doppler assessment of the utero-placental circulation in early pregnancy. Obstet Gynecol 1991;77:365–9.
11. Shih JC. Cesarean scar pregnancy: diagnosis with three-dimensional (3D) ultrasound and 3D power Doppler. Ultrasound Obstet Gynecol 2004;23:306–7.
12. Chou MM, Hwang JI, Tseng JJ, et al. Cesarean scar pregnancy: quantitative assessment of uterine neovascularization with 3-dimensional color power Doppler imaging and successful treatment with uterine artery embolization. Am J Obstet Gynecol 2004;190:866–8.
13. Vela G, Tulandi T. Cervical pregnancy: the importance of early diagnosis and treatment. J Minim Invasive Gynecol 2007;14:481.
14. Chazotte C, Cohen WR. Catastrophic complications of previous Cesarean section. Am J Obstet Gynecol 1990;163:738–42.

Evaluation of Suspected Fetal Skeletal Dysplasia for the Referring Physician

Monique Ho, MD

KEYWORDS

• Fetus • Osteochondrodysplasia • Prenatal diagnosis • Skeletal dysplasia • Ultrasonography

KEY POINTS

- Fetal skeletal abnormalities are common, and practitioners who perform prenatal ultrasonography will periodically encounter them.
- Prenatal evaluation of fetal skeletal dysplasia is complex, and the phenotype of even well-known disorders is often variable; ultrasonography can accurately predict the final diagnosis in only approximately 40% of cases.
- Prediction of perinatal lethality is good, approaching 98%, even if the ultimate diagnosis is incorrect.
- Many suspected fetal skeletal dysplasias cannot be confirmed with molecular genetic, histopathologic, or radiographic evaluation, and perinatal death is frequent. Counseling is ultimately based on the sonographic appearance for those whom diagnosis is not possible, making thorough ultrasonographic evaluation and prompt referral critical.

INTRODUCTION

The prevalence of skeletal dysplasias (osteochondrodysplasias) detectable prenatally or early in the neonatal period has been estimated at 1 in 5000 pregnancies, but is potentially higher.[1,2] These dysplasias are therefore common enough for the average referring prenatal sonologist to encounter on occasion, but not so frequent that they are familiar and easily recalled. As of the 2006 International Skeletal Dysplasia Society (ISDS) Nosology Group consensus statement there are 372 different conditions with genetic basis and significant skeletal involvement, classified into 37 groups of disorders.[3] For most referring centers, this means that the same skeletal dysplasia may never be encountered twice by a single practitioner. At least 50 of these disorders will have detectable findings prenatally,[4] but they may only be visible at gestational ages after the timing of a typical anatomic survey. In a prospective analysis of 500 consecutive referrals for abnormal skeletal findings by Krakow and colleagues[4] in 2008, the most common confirmed diagnoses were osteogenesis imperfecta type 2 (16%), thanatophoric dysplasia (12%), and achondrogenesis type 2 (6%). Achondroplasia is the most common nonlethal disorder at approximately 1 in 10,000 births (live or stillborn).[1,2]

We are only just beginning to explore the prenatal phenotype of genetic disorders, including those with major skeletal components, as we gain experience with early ultrasound imaging. Adaptation of Pediatric Radiology skeletal survey protocols[5] (using ultrasound input instead of x-rays) may become feasible as our understanding, as well as ultrasound equipment, improves. At the time of second-trimester ultrasound scan, the most immediate need is identification of those

Disclosures: The author has no conflict of interest to disclose.
Division of Maternal-Fetal Medicine, Department of OB/GYN, University of Rochester Medical Center, 601 Elmwood Avenue, Box #668, Rochester, NY 14642, USA
E-mail address: Monique_Ho@urmc.rochester.edu

Ultrasound Clin 8 (2013) 31–38
http://dx.doi.org/10.1016/j.cult.2012.08.012
1556-858X/13/$ – see front matter

fetuses with probable lethality. Two-dimensional ultrasonography remains the best diagnostic tool for this task, after improvements in resolution over the last 10 years. Three-dimensional (3D) imaging may add detail to facial dysmorphology or limb assessment, but does not seem to appreciably improve the diagnostic yield.[6]

FETAL SKELETAL DEVELOPMENT

Timing of Normal Skeletal Development

Primary ossification centers of the clavicle and mandible are visible by transvaginal sonography as early as 8 to 9 weeks of gestation, and 1 to 2 weeks later with the transabdominal approach.[7] The maxilla and long bones quickly follow in the 10th week, and most primary sites are visible by 15 weeks. Some primary centers appear late, such as 23 to 25 weeks for the superior pubic ramus, and the carpal bones will not be seen until well after birth. The secondary ossification centers become visible later in gestation, beginning with the calcaneus at 20 weeks, the distal femoral epiphysis after 32 weeks, and the proximal tibial epiphysis after 37 weeks.[8] Craniosynostosis is not detectable until after 16 to 18 weeks, even in the most severe manifestation of multiple synostoses (kleeblattschädel).[4]

Nosology of Abnormal Development

The 2006 ISDS Nosology[3] provides an at-a-glance orientation to the skeletal disorders as a whole, organizing them into 37 groups based on common genetic pathways (if known) or phenotypic hallmarks. Many of these relatively small groups can be further aggregated into 7 larger categories with features in common (**Box 1**).

Box 1
Categories of ISDS groups from 2006 consensus

Common affected protein or pathway (FGFR3, type II collagen)

Anatomic localization of radiographic changes (short ribs, metaphyseal changes)

Macroscopic global clinical findings (bent bones, dislocations)

Abnormalities of mineralization (increased or decreased density, stippling)

Lysosomal disorders with skeletal involvement

Disorganized skeletal components (exostoses, enchondromas)

Dysostoses (craniosynostoses, costovertebral dysostosis)

Elements of prenatal skeletal evaluation

Establishment of best gestational age by menstrual dates or first-trimester ultrasonography

Standard biometric measurements, fluid volume, and anatomic survey

External genitalia assessment

Axial skeleton

- Cranial contours in all planes including facial profile; 3D face is helpful if possible
- Axial, sagittal and coronal spine views
- Rib number, contour, and length
- Chest circumference at the level of the 4-chamber heart, with sagittal chest/abdomen view

Appendicular skeleton

- Measurement and contour of all long bones
- General assessment of joint mobility and contour
- Hands and feet (including all digits and angle of articulation with distal limb); 3D is helpful if possible
- Scapula coronal view

Indices

- Chest/abdominal circumference ratio (<0.6 suggests lethality)[9]
- Femur/abdominal circumference ratio (<0.16 suggests lethality)[9]
- Femur/foot ratio (normal ~1 regardless of gestational age)[9]

This organization assists the sonologist in development of a differential diagnosis, and therefore a loose prediction of a range of severity for on-the-spot counseling. Many of the diagnostic features will not be apparent prenatally, which is why accurate diagnosis is only possible in 40% of pregnancies, but if 1 or more groups are suspected counseling can be more specific.

SONOGRAPHIC FINDINGS SUGGESTING SKELETAL DYSPLASIA

A complete skeletal survey of the fetus may yield diagnostic abnormalities that would not otherwise be detected on routine screening views. An evaluation of mineralization, for example, may show poor calvarial bone ossification (**Fig. 1**) of osteogenesis imperfecta type 2. Sagittal view of the

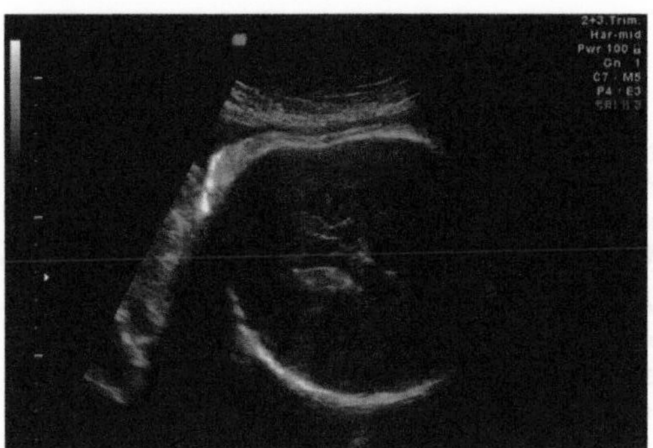

Fig. 1. Poor mineralization of fetal calvarium at 39 weeks' gestation in a fetus with osteogenesis imperfecta type 2. Deformation due to minimal transducer pressure is visible.

entire fetus (when possible in early gestation) allows visualization of alteration in body proportions such as the strikingly short thorax and protuberant abdomen of Jarcho-Levin syndrome (**Fig. 2**).

Proceeding to the axial skeleton, findings suggesting abnormality include abnormal cranial contours indicating craniosynostosis or glabellar bossing, midface hypoplasia with or without proptosis owing to shallow orbits, or microretrognathia. These features may appear nearly normal in early gestation, but become more striking over time, and vary in severity among individuals with the same disorder (**Fig. 3**). Vertebral anomalies with kyphoscoliosis may become apparent initially as the inability to image the entire spine in one sagittal

Sonographic appearance of the most common osteochondrodysplasias

Osteogenesis Imperfecta Type 2 (ISDS Decreased Bone Density Group)[10]

- Multiple evolving long bone and rib fractures typically visible in the second trimester, which is most commonly significantly deforming. Relatively normal hands and feet
- Poor bone mineralization, particularly striking in the calvarium, which may be easily depressed by transducer pressure
- May develop thickened nuchal translucency/fold or hydrops

Thanatophoric Dysplasia Type 1 or 2 (ISDS FGFR3 Group)[11]

- Striking thoracic hypoplasia visible in second trimester with bell-shaped thorax
- Platyspondyly, but relatively normal trunk length
- Severely short broad long bones, either bowed (type 1) or straight (type 2)
- Depressed nasal bridge and midface hypoplasia. Cloverleaf skull may be present, especially in type 2
- Normal bone density
- Frequent polyhydramnios

Achondrogenesis Type 2 (ISDS Type 2 Collagen Group)[12]

- Hydropic appearance in second trimester due to striking micromelia, barrel chest (vertically short thorax with short horizontal ribs), and protuberant abdomen
- Ossification of the spine, ischial bone, and pubic bone is completely absent or nearly so
- Midface hypoplasia and often cleft lip
- Polyhydramnios frequent

Campomelic Dysplasia (ISDS Bent Bones Dysplasias Group)[13,14]

- Small thorax but not always as visually striking as other lethal dysplasias, consistent with the reports of rare long-term survival; often with 11 pairs of ribs
- Bowing (with rare exceptions) of the femora and tibiae
- Male to female sex reversal in 60% to 70%
- Hypoplasia of the body of the scapula. This finding is also reported in Antley-Bixler syndrome, but the latter is distinguished by craniosynostosis and radiohumeral synostosis

Achondroplasia (ISDS FGFR3 Group)[15]

- Rhizomelic micromelia of all extremities, which may not be seen until the late second trimester, and short fingers giving "trident hand" appearance in third trimester
- Disproportionately large head and normal spine length, with midface hypoplasia and depressed nasal bridge; not as striking or early as lethal dysplasias
- No thoracic hypoplasia, fractures, or dislocations, and normal mineralization

Pearls and Pitfalls

Pearls

- *Probably lethal*: Chest/abdominal circumference ratio less than 0.6 and abnormal sagittal contour, especially if accompanied by the following: femur/abdominal circumference ratio less than 0.16, hydrops fetalis, severe polyhydramnios, visceral anomalies, craniosynostosis of multiple sutures (cloverleaf/kleeblattschädel skull), severe scapular hypoplasia, sex reversal
- *Probably abnormal; indeterminate severity*: Multiple long bones less than 5th percentile or greater than 3 standard deviations (SD) below mean without thoracic restriction and sure gestational age (particularly if the head circumference is >75th percentile), isolated craniosynostosis, nonspecific abnormalities of multiple skeletal elements, not meeting the above criteria for probable lethality
- Accuracy of prenatal prediction of lethality ~97%; prediction of diagnosis overall closer to 40%. Some disorders with perinatal lethality will be missed

Pitfalls

- The term skeletal dysplasia is a broad term describing a diverse group of hundreds of recognized disorders. Not all skeletal dysplasias are lethal, and many disorders have normal cognition. The high rate of perinatal death and significant developmental abnormalities, however, warrants cautious and thorough counseling by an experienced provider
- Some disorders with normal-appearing thoracic size are still lethal
- Gestational age may have a significant impact on the ability to detect some significant abnormalities, and diagnoses may be missed at the time of second-trimester anatomic survey (especially before ~18 weeks)
- False positives do exist[16]
- There is limited knowledge of the appearance and variability of specific rare disorders in early pregnancy. Phenotype at presentation may depend on gestational age and evolve over time
- Because of the high in utero and perinatal death rate, early completion of thorough sonographic evaluation is important, as the ultrasound visit may be the only opportunity. Image as much as you can, when you can.

or coronal plane (**Fig. 4**). Axial views of rib contour and length should encompass at least two-thirds of the chest circumference normally. Short, thick, gracile, missing, or abnormally angulated ribs may be apparent, and individual rib images as well as sagittal and coronal thoracic contour are helpful (**Fig. 5**). The conformation of the ilia, presence/absence of the ischia and pubic rami, and pelvic angles may narrow the differential as well, but can be more difficult to image.

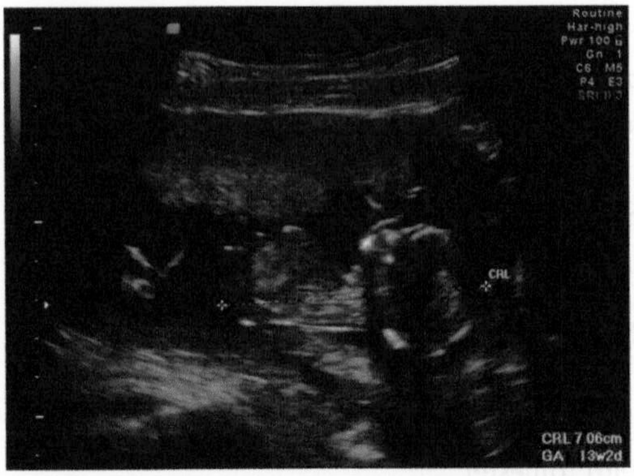

Fig. 2. Sagittal view of 13-week crown rump length of a fetus with Jarcho-Levin syndrome, demonstrating a strikingly short trunk and protuberant abdomen.

Views of the extremities, both as a whole to document joint position and proportion and by individual components to evaluate for bowing, fractures, absence, and/or shortening of long tubular bones (**Fig. 6**), should be systematic and thorough. Scapular hypoplasia is a particularly helpful finding if present.

PATHOPHYSIOLOGY

The pathophysiology of the osteochondrodysplasias is as varied as the disorders themselves. Of the 372 recognized disorders of skeletal development, 215 had causative mutations identified in 1 or more of 140 different genes, still leaving a substantial number that will not have an associated molecular diagnostic test available. To complicate matters further, different mutations within the same gene will have strikingly different clinical results (eg, the FGFR3 mutations

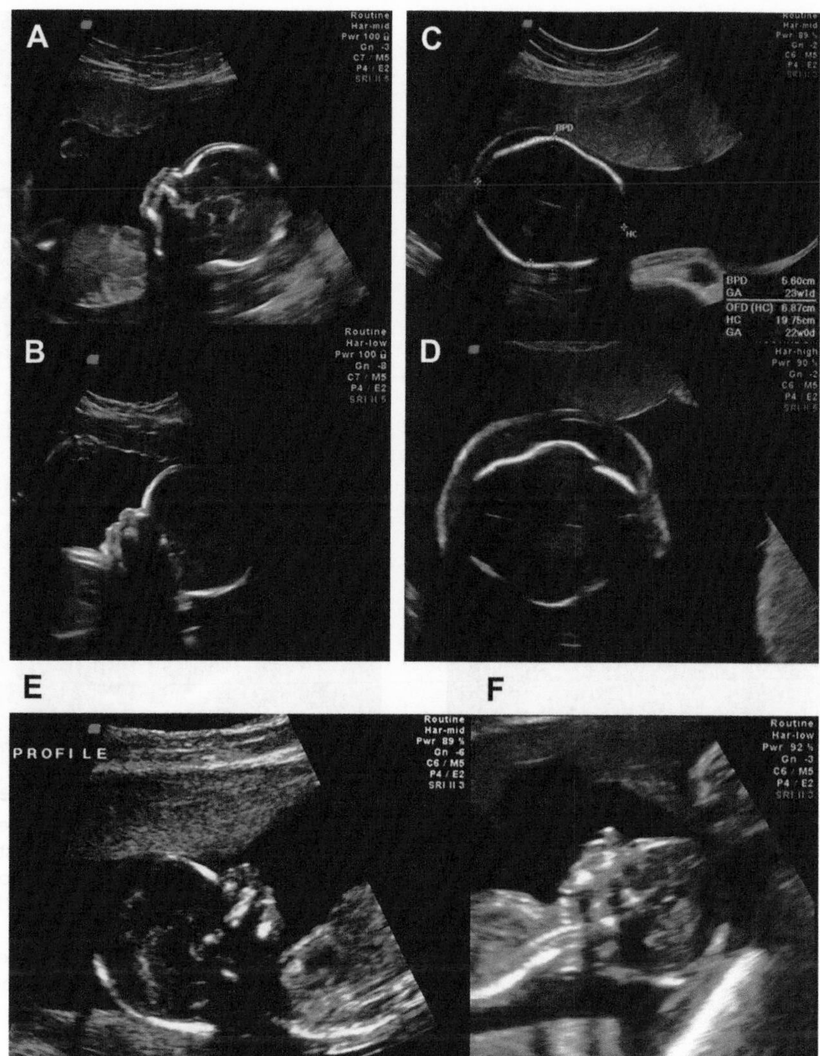

Fig. 3. Profile of a fetus with Apert syndrome at 18 weeks (*A*) and 28 weeks (*B*), demonstrating progressive glabellar bossing and midface hypoplasia. Axial views of the cranium showing abnormal contour of multiple craniosynostoses and hydrops at 22 weeks (*C*) and 25 weeks (*D*). (*E, F*) Siblings with Antley-Bixler syndrome at 16 weeks; both have early significant turricephaly and midface hypoplasia, but more severe micrognathia in *F* than in *E*.

responsible for thanatophoric dysplasia, achondroplasia, and hypochondroplasia). Also on occasion a single phenotype can be caused by mutations in multiple genes, causing different inheritance patterns in different families (eg, osteogenesis imperfecta type 2 can be associated with autosomal dominant mutations in COL1A1 or COL1A2, or with autosomal recessive inheritance of mutations in CRTAP or P3H1/LEPRE1).[3,17]

If attempting to find common ground for pathogenesis based on structural findings, the task is no easier. There are 40 distinct disorders with bowed femurs as a frequent occurrence, for example.[18] The causes range from relatively common FGFR3 gain-of-function mutations of thanatophoric dysplasia, or loss of SOX9 function in campomelic dysplasia, to rare pathology of type II collagen secretion resulting in Kniest dysplasia. It is possible to roughly group disorders by the general component of bone development affected, such as skeletal morphogenesis, chondrocyte differentiation and enchondral bone formation, osteoblast differentiation and function, or extracellular matrix formation, as the pathways involved for each are relatively distinct.[17] However, there is enough overlap in components

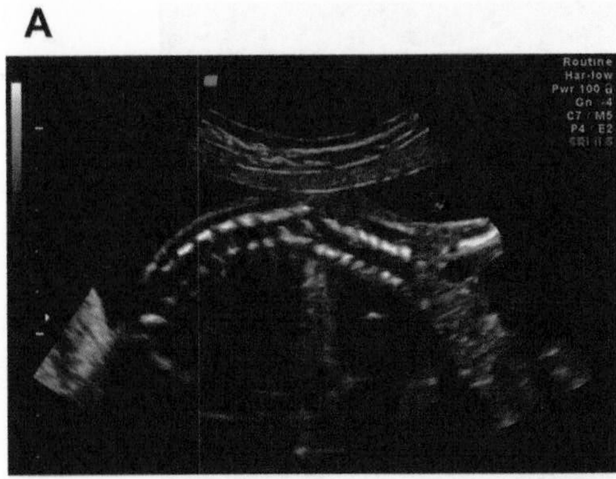

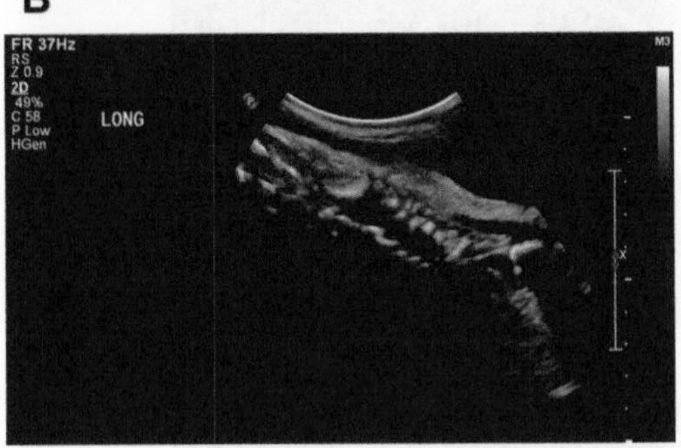

Fig. 4. Vertebral anomalies and sharply angulated kyphoscoliosis in the same fetus at 20 weeks' (*A*) and 33 weeks' (*B*) gestation.

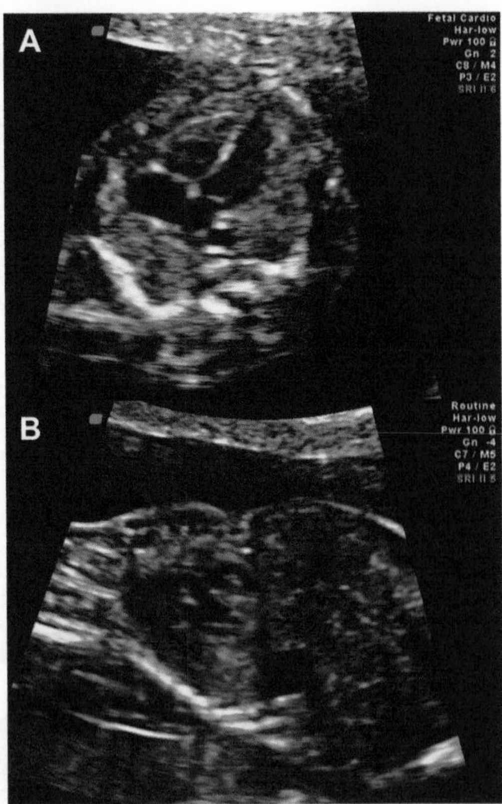

Fig. 5. (*A*)Axial view of the thorax in a fetus with thanatophoric dysplasia type 1, demonstrating small chest circumference relative to the normal cardiac size, short angulated ribs, and skin thickening of hydrops. (*B*) Longitudinal thorax and abdomen in the same fetus showing severe thoracic restriction and comparatively large protuberant abdomen.

What the referring physician needs to know

Triggers for more Comprehensive Evaluation and Referral

- Small chest circumference with abnormal thoracic contour on sagittal view
- Long bone measurements at less than 5th percentile or less than 3 SD for gestational age, or absence of any skeletal element
- Any abnormalities of cranial or individual bone contour
- Abnormal limb contour or mobility

Range of Severity and Inheritance

- Virtually all modes of inheritance are accounted for in this broad group of disorders, and phenotypes from normal except orthopedic accommodations, to prenatally lethal are represented. Narrowing down the differential to a particular nosologic category (eg, bent bones or hypomineralization) likewise narrows the suspected range of severity to assist initial counseling
- Prediction of perinatal lethality by small thoracic circumference and abnormal sagittal contour in the second trimester is highly accurate; however, assignment of a particular diagnosis (particularly for nonlethal disorders) based on prenatal findings is correct in less than half of patients, and some lethal diagnoses will be missed

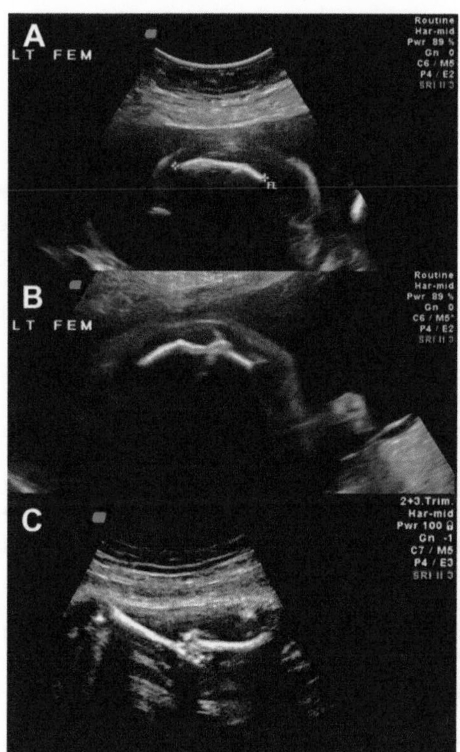

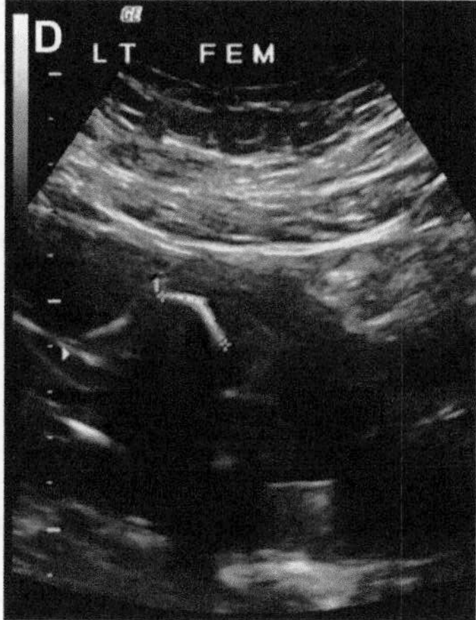

Fig. 6. Change in femur fracture appearance over time, at 20 weeks (*A*) and 28 weeks (*B*) in a fetus with osteogenesis imperfecta type 2, and an unrelated fetus with the same disorder at 39 weeks (*C*). (*D*) If occurring at midshaft, fractures can be difficult to distinguish from the angulated femur of thanatophoric dysplasia type 1.

and variation in downstream effect of pathway alterations to ensure that for the average provider this is not a practical mnemonic.

SUMMARY

Fetal osteochondrodysplasias are a relatively common problem that all prenatal sonologists will likely run into eventually. Such a diverse group of disorders makes prenatal assignment of a specific diagnosis difficult even for world experts in the field, although prediction of perinatal lethality based on the aforementioned criteria is good. It is clearly important to recognize and refer affected pregnancies in timely fashion not only to preserve all management options before viability, but for delivery planning for lethal or nonlethal diagnoses alike. For example, many newborns with midface hypoplasia or even mild thoracic restriction have upper airway obstruction or other neonatal issues that require immediate support, preparation, and specialists.

Referring physicians play a vital role in triage and initial counseling, as well as in supplying images, movie clips, and measurements to assist the referral center. Because there is a high rate of death in utero or immediately after delivery, the pattern of change over time may provide important diagnostic clues to the pathologist, and this can allow for better counseling regarding future pregnancies.

Gestational age has a significant impact on detection; for example, shortening of long bones for nonlethal disorders may not reliably be present until after 18 weeks.[4] In a large Swedish study of ultrasound screening for structural anomalies comparing a planned single evaluation at 12 to 14 weeks with one at 15 to 22 weeks, only 50% of the osteochondrodysplasias were suspected prenatally in the early group compared with 80% in those examined later.[19] This difference did not achieve statistical significance because of low numbers, but it makes sense that those in the 15- to 22-week group would have a more strikingly abnormal appearance, owing to the cumulative effect over time of divergence from the normal rate of growth. Understanding of these principles will, it is hoped, provide the referring sonologist with the necessary tools to maximize diagnostic accuracy and aid patient counseling.

REFERENCES

1. Rasmussen S, Bieber F, Benacerraf B, et al. Epidemiology of osteochondrodysplasias: changing trends due to advances in prenatal diagnosis. Am J Med Genet 1996;61:49–58.
2. Orioli I, Castilla E, Barbosa-Neto J. The birth prevalence rates for the skeletal dysplasias. J Med Genet 1986;23:328–32.
3. Superti-Furga A, Unger S, the Nosology Group of the International Skeletal Dysplasia Society. Nosology and classification of genetic skeletal disorders: 2006 revision. Am J Med Genet A 2007;143:1–18.
4. Krakow D, Alanay Y, Rimoin L, et al. Evaluation of prenatal-onset osteochondrodysplasias by ultrasonography: a retrospective and prospective analysis. Am J Med Genet A 2008;146(15):1917–24.
5. Offiah A, Hall C. Radiological diagnosis of the constitutional disorders of bone. As easy as A, B, C? Pediatr Radiol 2003;33:153–61.
6. Krakow D, Williams J, Poehl M, et al. Use of three-dimensional ultrasound imaging in the diagnosis of prenatal-onset skeletal dysplasias. Ultrasound Obstet Gynecol 2003;21:467–72.
7. van Zalen-Sprock R, Brons J, van Vugt J, et al. Ultrasonographic and radiologic visualization of the developing embryonic skeleton. Ultrasound Obstet Gynecol 1997;9:392–7.
8. Olsen ØE, Lie RT, Lachman RS, et al. Ossification sequence in infants who die during the perinatal period: population-based references. Radiology 2002;225:240–4.
9. Krakow D, Lachman R, Rimoin D. Guidelines for the prenatal diagnosis of fetal skeletal dysplasias. Genet Med 2009;11(2):127–33.
10. Spranger JW, Brill PW, Poznanski A. Osteogenesis imperfecta, type IIA and IIC. Bone dysplasias; an atlas of genetic disorders of skeletal development. 2nd edition. New York: Oxford University Press; 2002. p. 436–9.
11. Spranger JW, Brill PW, Poznanski A. Thanatophoric dysplasia, types 1 and 2. In: Bone dysplasias; an atlas of genetic disorders of skeletal development. 2nd edition. New York: Oxford University Press; 2002. p. 3–6.
12. Spranger JW, Brill PW, Poznanski A. Achondrogenesis, type II. Bone dysplasias; an atlas of genetic disorders of skeletal development. 2nd edition. New York: Oxford University Press; 2002. p. 11–2.
13. Spranger JW, Brill PW, Poznanski A. Campomelic dysplasia. Bone dysplasias; an atlas of genetic disorders of skeletal development. 2nd edition. New York: Oxford University Press; 2002. p. 41–6.
14. Mortier G, Rimoin D, Lachman R. The scapula as a window to the diagnosis of skeletal dysplasias. Pediatr Radiol 1997;27:447–51.
15. Spranger JW, Brill PW, Poznanski A. Achondroplasia. In: Bone dysplasias; an atlas of genetic disorders of skeletal development. 2nd edition. New York: Oxford University Press; 2002. p. 83–9.
16. Parilla B, Leeth E, Kambich M, et al. Antenatal detection of skeletal dysplasias. J Ultrasound Med 2003;22:255–8.
17. Olsen B, Reginato A, Wang W. Bone development. Annu Rev Cell Dev Biol 2000;16:191–220.
18. Alanay Y, Krakow D, Rimoin D, et al. Angulated femurs and the skeletal dysplasias: experience of the international skeletal dysplasia registry (1988-2006). Am J Med Genet A 2007;143:1159–68.
19. Saltvedt S, Almström H, Kublickas M, et al. Detection of malformations in chromosomally normal fetuses by routine ultrasound at 12 or 18 weeks of gestation—a randomised controlled trial in 39,572 pregnancies. BJOG 2006;113:664–74.

Effects of Obesity on Obstetric Ultrasound Imaging

Loralei L. Thornburg, MD

KEYWORDS

• Ultrasound scan • Obesity • Anatomic evaluation • First-trimester screening • Genetic sonogram • Anomaly • Nuchal translucency

KEY POINTS

- Obesity, especially morbid obesity, limits the ability to complete screening in pregnancy.
- Obese patients are at higher risk for fetal anomalies and failure to detect anomalies before birth than their normal-weight counterparts.
- Birth weight prediction in obese patients by the gestation-adjusted prediction method seems to be accurate and allows evaluation of the fetus at a gestational age when visualization is improved.

INTRODUCTION

Obesity is increasing worldwide, with most of the industrialized world having obesity rates of 20%–30% in the adult population and some selected populations, such as the southern Pacific, reporting obesity rates of 44%–80%.[1,2] Obesity is defined as a body mass index (BMI) of greater than 30 and is generally divided into classes, with class I consisting of BMI of 30.0–34.9 kg/m^2, class II BMI of 35.0–39.9 kg/m^2, and class III BMI of $\geq$40 kg/m^2. Class III has also been called *extreme obesity* and represents body weights 50%–100% higher than ideal.[1,3] According to the World Health Organization, "(obesity) is now so common that it is replacing the more traditional concerns…as one of the most significant contributors to ill health."[1] Weight, age, and parity all tend to increase in concert, and obesity can lead to increase medical concerns; therefore, the obese woman often tends to have additional medical concerns and may be of advanced maternal age.[4,5]

The ability to penetrate an obese patient can be limited in ultrasound scan; therefore, understanding the limitations of visualization in this population is important for the clinician counseling patients regarding their pregnancy risks. Obesity is also a major risk factor for numerous obstetric complications and may limit a clinician's ability to assess the health of the fetus by ultrasound scan.

GENERAL APPROACH TO ULTRASOUND IN THE OBESE PATIENT

There is no question that with increased depth of penetration, there is increased absorption and dispersion of the sound waves, such that the reflected signal is distorted and weakened, resulting in backscatter and an increased noise-to-signal ratio.[6] Therefore, when performing ultrasound scan on the obese patient, the sonographer must take into account the altered habitus and plan accordingly. In general, the sonographer should make an effort to find and use the best acoustic windows for a woman's habitus. Adjusting approaches to improve ultrasound visualization has been suggested, most with little prospective data (**Box 1**). In general, abdominal adiposity tends to cluster centrally below the umbilicus and above pubis, with little at the inferior abdomen, umbilicus, or laterally.[6] Therefore, for some morbidly obese women, visualization may

Disclosures: None.
Conflicts of interest: None.

Division of Maternal Fetal Medicine, Department of OB/GYN, University of Rochester Medical Center, University of Rochester, 601 Elmwood Avenue Box 668, Rochester, NY 14642, USA
E-mail address: Loralei_thornburg@urmc.rochester.edu

Ultrasound Clin 8 (2013) 39–47
http://dx.doi.org/10.1016/j.cult.2012.08.013
1556-858X/13/$ – see front matter

ultrasound.theclinics.com

Box 1
Tips for scanning obese patients to improve visualization

- Use of the lateral, inferior, or periumbilical regions, because abdominal adiposity tends to cluster centrally below the umbilicus and above pubis
- Retraction of skin apron to allow visualization within the superpubic fold
- Rolling patient onto her side
- Making use of the iliac fossa
- Use of a narrow probe or even the transvaginal probe within a deep umbilicus
- Use of the maternal bladder as a window and to raise the uterus out of the pelvis
- Combined transvaginal/transabdominal approach with the transvaginal probe used to elevate the uterus out of the pelvis, and the transabdominal approach to visualize the fetus
- Upright scanning with the patient sitting to displace adipose inferiorly
- Transvaginal assessment for those fetal parts near the cervix
- Use of harmonic imaging, spatial compounding, and speckle reduction filters

Data from Paladini D. Sonography in obese and overweight pregnant women: clinical, medicolegal and technical issues. Ultrasound Obstet Gynecol 2009;33:720–9; Bromley B, Shipp TD, Mitchell, et al. Tricks for obtaining a nuchal translucency measurement on the fetus in a difficult position. J Ultrasound Med 2010;29:1261–4; Thornburg LL. Antepartum obstetrical complications associated with obesity. Semin Perinatol 2011;35:317–23.

be best underneath the pannus at the pubis, whereas for others, the skin apron may be relaxed and inferiorly displaced enough that the depth of penetration is actually better above the fold. If an under-the-pannus approach is taken, the sonographer may need to request help from the patient or family in holding or retracting her abdomen to allow hand movements once within the fold. Additionally, care should be taken to fully dry this area after completion, because it is prone to breakdown with increased wetness. Rolling a patient onto her side may improve visualization (**Fig. 1**), as can using the iliac fossa, which generally also has less adipose tissue (**Fig. 2**). Prior abdominal scarring from cesarean delivery or multiple gestation, both more frequent in obese patients, can also decrease visualization.[4,6]

For some women, the umbilicus may provide a window, and a narrow probe or even transvaginal probe within a deep umbilicus may improve visualization. However, the angles and mobility of the probe are limited. Using the maternal bladder as a window is critical, especially in the first trimester, and in later pregnancy, a full bladder may serve to raise the uterus out of the pelvis and move the fetal target closer to the surface of the maternal abdomen.[6] Other suggested strategies include combining transvaginal/transabdominal approach, using the transvaginal probe to elevate the uterus out of the pelvis, and the transabdominal approach to visualize the fetus.[7] Upright scanning with the patient sitting may further displace the adipose inferiorly and provide acoustic windows, and for those fetal parts that are near the cervix, transvaginal assessment may also be valuable.[8]

Visualization may be limited even with the best equipment, and scanning of the obese patient can represent a physical challenge to the sonographer, with the literature suggesting that scanning obese patients contributes to injury.[9,10] Making sure that the physical environment is not contributing to sonographer burden is important (**Box 2**), and ideally alterations should include higher stools and high-rated, motorized patient beds so that patients can be easily positioned and repositioned as the scan proceeds. If patients lack mobility, ultrasound scans can be performed in motorized wheelchairs and scooters, especially if these can be reclined, to avoid staff having to transfer patients. If a transvaginal approach is used, the weight rating of the bed should be checked against the patient weight, because if a morbidly obese patient is placed in stirrups on an unbolted, underrated bed, weight readjustment can cause the bed to tip. The larger the patient, the pressure a sonographer will have to apply over likely a prolonged period of time is higher, and this prolonged orthopedic strain likely increases the risk for injury.[6,9,10] Therefore, sonographers may need to adjust their body position frequently or, in the case of particularly long ultrasound examinations, such as an anatomic survey in twins on a morbidly obese patient, change operators midway through the examination.

Ultrasound equipment should have optimized obesity and penetration settings to aid in completing scans more comfortably and quickly, which may help reduce the risks of sonographer injury because of needing to use less pressure and time to adequately visualize. Harmonic imaging (**Figs. 3** and **4**) and spatial compounding and speckle reduction filters can markedly improve the visualization in these women and should be

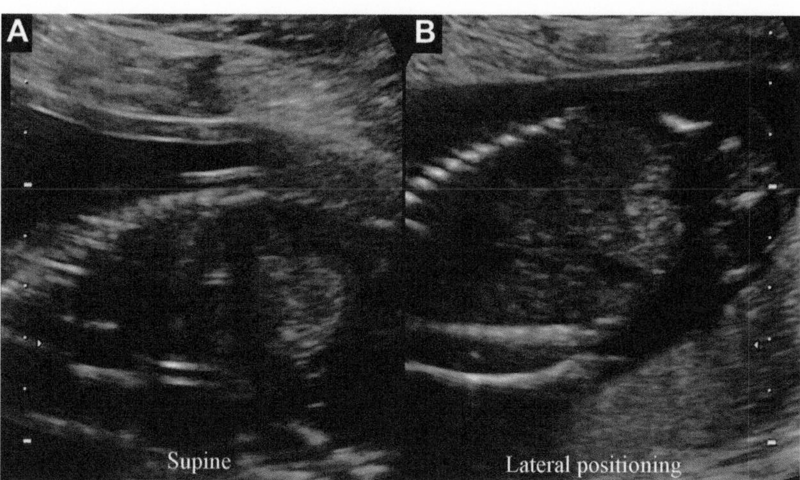

Fig. 1. Lateral positioning. The supine position (*A*) may have decreased visualization compared to lateral positioning (*B*), which can allow use of the thinner lateral abdomen and shift a pannus away from the fetal parts. In the image obtained in the lateral position (*B*), there is markedly better visualization of the fetal abdomen, chest contours, and bladder without changing any other settings.

part of this "obesity" setting (**Fig. 5**).[6,11] Doppler imaging may also help with visualization of cardiac inflows and outflows.[6] Regardless, before any imaging, the patient should be counseled regarding the technical limitations, from obesity and other medical conditions, and the increased risk of undiagnosed fetal anomalies.[6,8,12]

Obesity and First-Trimester Screening

As obesity increases with maternal age, early and accurate screening ultrasound scan for aneuploidy screening is important. Although first-trimester screening is offered to all women, there is a failure rate associated with this test. The First and Second Trimester Screening (FaSTER) trial had a failure rate of only 7.1% for nuchal translucency (NT) measurement.[13] However, other studies have found higher failure rates outside of the study setting, with Wax and colleagues[14] showing a 20% NT failure rate on first attempt among all comers (taking into account that some patients will be referred at an inappropriate gestational age or have a nonviable pregnancy), which is

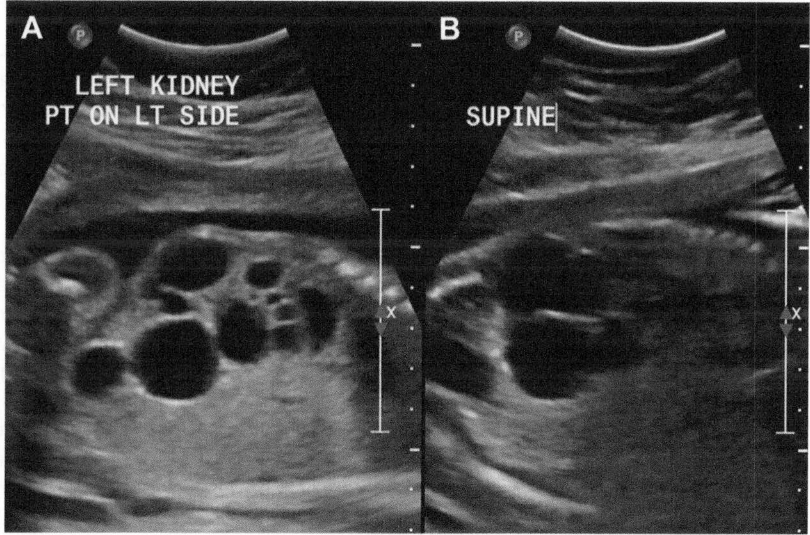

Fig. 2. Use of the iliac fossa. Because adiposity tends to cluster in the central lower abdomen, using the iliac fossa (*A*) where there is less thickness may improve visualization. In visualizing this multicystic abnormal fetal kidney, the views obtained through the central abdomen (*B*) lack the clarity of those images obtained through the lateral iliac fossa (*A*), where individual cysts become clearly visible.

Box 2
Alterations to care for obese patients in the ultrasound environment

Create an accessible and comfortable office environment

- Sturdy, armless chairs and high, firm sofas in waiting and examination rooms, because obese patients often have obese family members
- Extra-large examination gowns or sheets to provide adequate coverage

Use medical equipment that can accurately assess patients

- Sturdy, wide examination tables bolted to the floor to prevent tipping
- Stool or step with handles to help patients get on the examination table
- Hydraulic beds that easily allow patients to easily get on and off the table

Reduce patient fears about weight

- Avoid the term *obesity*—many patients may be more comfortable with terms such as *difficulties with weight* or *being overweight*
- Only ask about weight or weigh patient when medically appropriate and do so in private

Protect the safety of the ultrasound staff

- Examination chairs for sonographers with adjustment to support arms and allow position changes
- Rotation of sonographers during ultrasound examination if particularly long or difficult
- Maximization of settings to minimize time and effort required to obtain images
- Use of assist devices and beds that easily allow patients to be repositioned to improve imaging

Data from World Health Organization. Obesity: preventing and managing the global epidemic. WHO technical report series 894. Geneva (Switzerland): World Health Organization, 2000; Paladini D. Sonography in obese and overweight pregnant women: clinical, medicolegal and technical issues. Ultrasound Obstet Gynecol 2009;33:720–9; Thornburg LL. Antepartum obstetrical complications associated with obesity. Semin Perinatol 2011;35:317–23.

more of real world failure number. Repeated attempts did seem to improve completion rates to at least 84% and as high as 97% when removing no-shows.[14]

For obese women, the completion rates for NT screening seem to be much lower. The largest series on NT failure rates among obese women suggest that obese women are less likely to be able to complete NT screening ultrasound scans, even with the addition of extra time and repeat assessments (**Table 1**), and this clearly trends with class of obesity.[15] Several other studies have also found that the time per patient is longer with obese patients for NT screening, adding to the burden of sonographer work.[15,16] Obesity also increases the need for transvaginal assessment for the NT (23% vs 41% in obese patients), and also reduces the likelihood of visualizing the nasal bone (NB), with 97% of normal-weight patients having adequate visualization of the NB compared with 87.3% of obese patients.[16]

This is particularly important when patients are trying to decide on the use of invasive testing techniques. Although the data suggest that most obese women who desire NT screening will be able to obtain it, there is a stiller higher risk of NT screen failure. This is especially true with the morbidly class III obese patient, in whom, even after repeated attempts, greater than10% will fail to have an NT measurement obtained.[15] These patients should be counseled before the NT assessment and should be prepared for a longer examination, high likelihood of transvaginal assessment, and the possibility of repeat visit.[14–16] Even in the best of circumstances, they should be prepared for the possibility of having to await second-trimester screening.

Obesity and Second-Trimester Genetic Sonogram

For many ultrasound units, the initial aneuploidy risk assessment is determined by maternal age, serum analytes, and NT screening and then is further tailored at the time of second-trimester screening ultrasound scan by the use of soft-marker assessment. These findings vary in their association with aneuploidy and can help guide the use of invasive fetal testing. Importantly, the absence of these markers is also used to reassure many patients with borderline positive screening. Several studies have looked at the genetic sonogram among obese patients and found poor completion rates. Tsai and colleagues[17] showed that on the first attempt at soft marker screening, 60% of normal-weight women completed the examination compared with only 49% of obese women, with the rates decreasing to as low as 38% in class III obese women. Even after repeated attempts, normal-weight women had significantly higher rates not completing the genetic screening

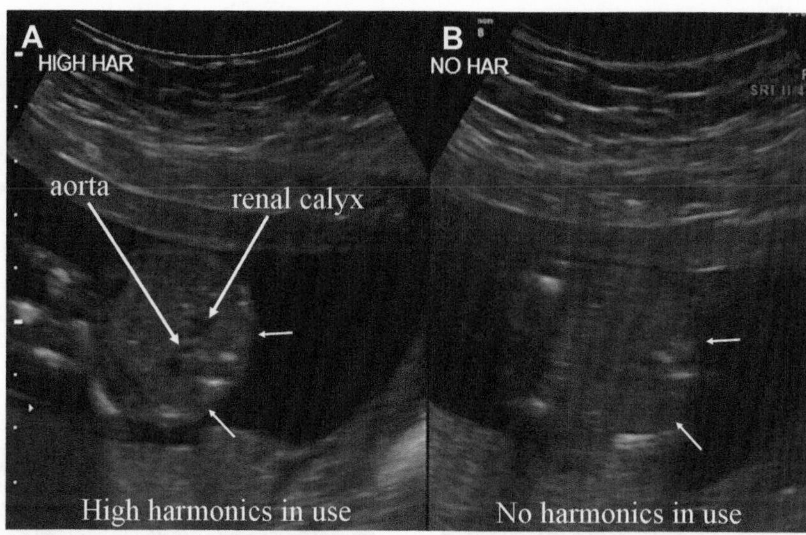

Fig. 3. Use of harmonics. Use of harmonics may improve visualization of fetal structures, such as the fetal kidneys in this image. When harmonics are in use (*A*), the kidneys (*arrows*) are much better visualized, and the renal calyxes and even aorta become visible, which are not visible without harmonics (*B*).

sonogram, with 63% completing the assessment compared with 55% of obese women (47% of class III obese). Additionally, even in women completing the scan, the rates of finding some markers, including short humerus and femur, varied by class of obesity, suggesting that visualization was likely suboptimal.[17] The FaSTER data showed similar results, with obese women having a lower sensitivity (22% vs 32%) of the genetic sonogram, a higher false-negative rate (78% vs 68%), and higher missed diagnosis rate compared with normal-weight patients.[18] If an obese patient is using ultrasound soft marker screening as her only screening method to guide the need for invasive testing, she should be aware of the limitations. Conversely, if the lack of soft marker findings is being used to reassure an obese patient with abnormal screening, the ultrasound detection limits for these should also be discussed.

Obesity and Second-Trimester Assessment For Anomalies

Obesity is clearly associated with an increased risk of fetal anomalies. Defects of the neural tube are markedly increased with reported odds ratios (OR) of 1.7–3.5 for spina bifida and 7.3 for encephaloceles, with these risks rising even higher when obesity is complicated by diabetes.[19–25] Cardiac defects are also increased, with ORs of 1.4–2.0 over those of the normal-weight population.[20–22] However, for some specific cardiac anomalies, the risks may be even higher, such as abnormalities of the great arteries (OR, 4.4) and common arterial truck defects (OR, 6.3) over those of the normal-weight population.[25] These data suggest that adequate visualization of the fetal heart and spine in obese patients is of particular concern.

However, maternal BMI has been noted by multiple authors to limit the ability to visualize fetal structures in the second trimester, and therefore limit ultrasound-based risk screening in this population.[26–30] In 2 of the largest studies, Dashe and colleagues[27] (>10,000 women) and Thornburg and colleagues[29] (>6500 women) noted similar results, with completion rates of anatomic ultrasound decreasing as maternal BMI increased (**Table 2**). Both also noted a poor ability to complete the survey at the first attempt, with Dashe and colleagues noting a completion rate of 50% on the first attempt for obese patients, while Thornburg and colleagues noted a first attempt completion rate of 41% for class I, 23% for class II and 17% for class III obese patients.[27,29] During these ultrasound anatomic evaluations, the spine and heart were the structures most likely to be poorly visualized.[29,31] As discussed earlier, these are also the structures most likely to be anomalous in the obese patient, especially if there is associated diabetes.[21,22] Rates of completion of the cardiac anatomy, including outflows, seem to be particularly limited, with the data from Thornburg and colleagues[29] showing that only 72% of patients with class III obesity ever completed the 4-chamber view (64% right outflow, 70% left outflow) even after repeated attempts, compared with a 91% completion of the 4-chamber view (89% right outflow, 90% left outflow) in normal-weight patients. Hendler and colleagues[31] also showed a high suboptimal visualization rate

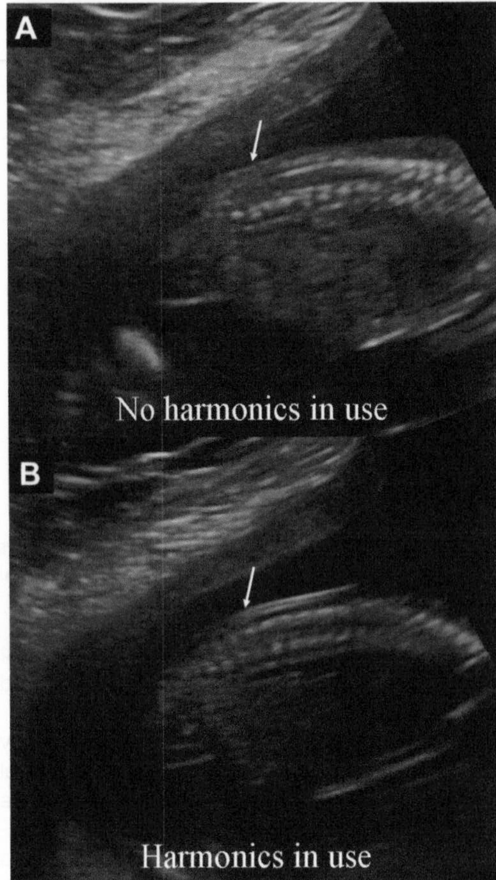

Fig. 4. Use of harmonics to visualize the spine. Compared to images without harmonics (*A*), use of harmonics (*B*) improves the visualization of skin line and sacral spine (*arrow*) over the images obtained without harmonics (*A*), which is important, as obese patients are at high risk for neural tube defects.

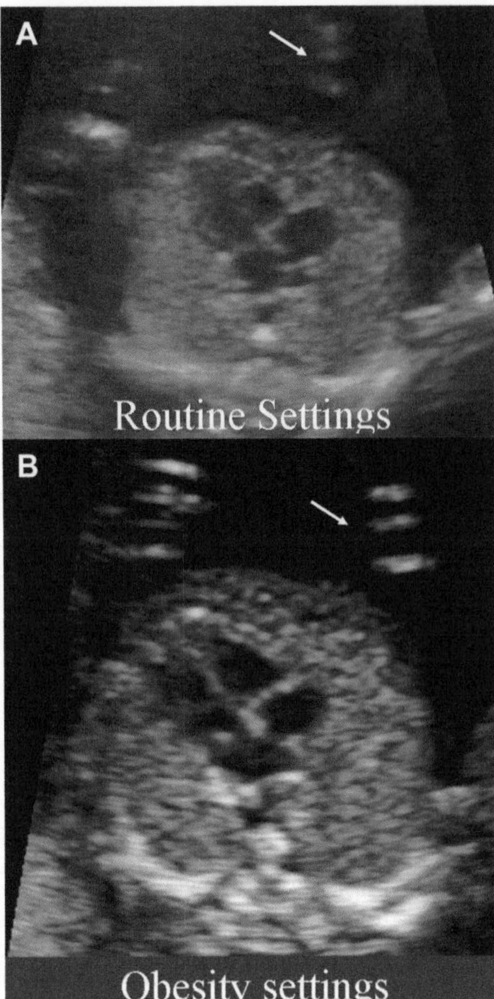

Fig. 5. Obesity-specific settings. Images without obesity-specific settings (*A*) lack clarity compared to those that, use obese specific settings (*B*) which include the use of harmonics and spatial compounding and speckle reduction filters can markedly improve visualization over standard settings (*A*). Note also the improved visualization of the umbilical cord (*arrows*).

for obese women for cardiac anatomy, with 18.7% of normal-weight women having suboptimally visualized fetal cardiac structures compared with 29.6% of class I, 39% of class II, and 49.3% of class III obese women, and other studies have had similar results.[31,32] Both studies also showed poor visualization of the craniospinal structures, with Hendler and colleagues[31] reporting suboptimal visualization in 29.5% of normal-weight women compared with 36.8% of class I, 43.3% of class II, and 53.4% of class III.

Multiple strategies have been suggested to improve visualization in the obese gravida, especially for the heart and spine. Improvement of ultrasound equipment did not seem to improve completion rates for these critical structures in an earlier study Hendler and colleagues,[33] but this study was completed before some of the more recent technologic advances. Because of this, other investigators have questioned this conclusion and suggested that harmonic imaging as well as spatial compounding and speckle reduction filters may markedly improve the visualization of cardiac views (see Figs. 2–4).[6] Senior sonographers are also more likely to obtain adequate visualization.[26] Repeat examination seems to decrease the rate of suboptimal visualization and improve completion rate.[28,29]

The timing of examination has also been evaluated to attempt to improve visualization. Transvaginal assessment for an early anatomic assessment between 12 and 14 weeks has been suggested as the optimal time to visualize extremities and hands, as there are reports that limb

Table 1
Failure rates for NT ultrasound scan by BMI class

	Normal Weight	All Obese	Obese		
			Class I	Class II	Class III
First attempt	2.2%	9.7%	5.4%	8.8%	22.7%
Repeated attempt	1.6%	6.6%	3.9%	6.7%	13.5%

Data from Thornburg LL, Mulconry M, Post A, et al. Fetal nuchal translucency thickness evaluation in the overweight and obese gravida. Ultrasound Obstet Gynecol 2009;33:665–9.

reduction defects are higher in obese patients, with then a follow-up assessment for the remainder of the anatomy later in pregnancy.[6,22] However, to minimize visits, other studies have suggested delaying the initial assessment to 18– 20 weeks to improve completion rates.[29,34] One small study (245 obese women) suggested delaying until 22–24 weeks to further improve completion, as they noted a single examination completion rate of 92% at this gestational age compared with completion rate of 88%–89% at 18–22 weeks.[26] Both of the larger studies addressing this question have found 18–20 to be superior. Lantz and colleagues,[34] in a study of 1444 women (448 obese), concluded that the 18- to 19-week window was optimal with completion rates of 68% at 18–20 and 76% at 20–22 weeks compared with 46% at 15–18 and 65% at 22–24 weeks. Thornburg and colleagues,[29] in a study of 7140 women (1952 obese), found that completion rates improve for each class of obesity until 20 weeks then decline. Therefore, given the preferred gestational age for aneuploidy testing and the legal limits of pregnancy termination for anomalies, 18–20 weeks is likely a better window. Regardless, patients should be aware that they are likely to require additional imaging options, including repeat visits, position changes, and use of transvaginal assessment.

After completion of the anatomic survey, there remains a substantial residual risk of anomaly in the obese patient. The most recent data suggest that routine and targeted ultrasound scan has a detection rate at least 20% lower in obese compared with normal-weight women (**Table 3**), giving a residual risk of anomaly of 0.4% for normal-weight patients, and 1% for obese patients.[12] Even when referred for targeted ultrasound scan because of a prior abnormal ultrasound scan or high-risk indication, detection rates are markedly lower for obese women (see **Table 3**).[12] The detection rate was also lower in pregestational diabetic women (38%) compared with 88% in those without diabetes but with other high-risk indications.[12] In the FaSTER study, detection of cardiac anomalies was 21.6% in normal-weight women compared with 8.3% in obese women with a much higher false-positive rate in obese women (91.7% obese vs 78.4% normal weight women).[18] The OR for sonographic detection of anomalies in obese patients was 0.7.[18] Given these data, the obese patient should likely be made aware of the increased residual risk of anomaly despite normal ultrasound screening.[6,12,29]

Fetal Weight Estimation in the Obese Gravida

Obese patients are at risk for macrosomia, especially if they also have excessive weight gain or diabetes, with maternal obesity alone giving at

Table 2
Completion of anatomic ultrasound evaluation (multiple attempts)

Type of Ultrasound Survey	Normal Weight[a]	Overweight	Obese		
			Class I	Class II	Class III
Basic (10 structures)	72%	68%	57%	41%	30%
Basic (12 structures)	79%	76%	72%	61%	49%
Comprehensive (18 structures)	43%	40%	38%	41%	31%

[a] Dashe et al. included underweight patients within the normal-weight category.

Adapted from Dashe JS, McIntire DD, Twickler DM. Maternal obesity limits the ultrasound evaluation of fetal anatomy. J Ultrasound Med 2009;28:1025–30; and Thornburg LL, Miles K, Ho M, et al. Fetal anatomic evaluation in the overweight and obese gravida. Ultrasound Obstet Gynecol 2009;33:670–5.

Table 3
Detection of fetal anomalies in the obese gravida

			Obese		
	Normal Weight	Overweight	Class I	Class II	Class III
Standard ultrasound	66%	49%	48%	42%	25%
Targeted Ultrasound	97%	91%	75%	88%	75%

Data from Dashe JS, McIntire DD, Twickler DM. Effect of maternal obesity on the ultrasound detection of anomalous fetuses. Obstet Gynecol 2009;113:1001–7.

least a 2-fold increased risk of macrosomia.[35] Prediction of macrosomia may be especially difficult in obese women given their habitus and the inability to accurately assess the fetal weight through Leopold's maneuvers, fundal heights, or other clinical assessments. There are data that indicate intrapartum and late pregnancy estimates of weight may be less accurate than those done earlier (34–36 weeks) in pregnancy and then projected forward, known as the *gestational adjusted prediction* (GAP) method.[36] The GAP method extrapolates estimated fetal weights forward using Brenner's median fetal weight curves and has the advantage in the obese gravida of measuring the fetal weight when the infant is higher in the pelvis, making head measurement easier, and when the amniotic fluid volume is greater, making acoustic windows better. There is evidence that fetal weight estimations using Hadlock's formulas may become less accurate when fetal weights are greater than 4500 g, a more common occurrence in the obese, especially obese diabetic woman at late term, giving additional value to estimating the fetal weight earlier in the pregnancy.[37] The GAP method has also been shown to be accurate in both diabetic and obese women.[38,39] However, there seems to be a tendency to overestimate weight in class I and II obese women and underestimate those with class III obesity. Regardless, the systematic and random error of the GAP method suggests that for obese patients, this method would predict birth weight within 20% over 90% of the time regardless of the obesity class.[38] Importantly, this method also had an excellent negative predictive value (>90%) for exclusion of macrosomia.[38] Regardless, all methods of fetal weight estimation have an associated error; therefore, clinical assessment of the entire patient picture is imperative.

SUMMARY

Obese women require additional considerations when planning the ultrasound approach. Typically, they require additional time, effort, and ultrasound examinations than their normal-weight counterparts. Screening options may be limited, and there is a higher risk for a missed diagnosis for all prenatal sonographic approaches. There is also a risk that anatomic evaluations cannot be completed, and even when completed, will have a higher residual risk for fetal anomalies. Birth weight prediction and following fetal growth will also be more difficult. Therefore, the clinician must partner with patients to assure that they understand the risks and benefits of different approaches and the technical limitations from obesity and other associated medical conditions on ultrasound evaluations.

REFERENCES

1. World Health Organization. Obesity: preventing and managing the global epidemic. WHO technical report series 894. Geneva (Switzerland): World Health Organization; 2000.
2. Popkin BM, Doak CM. The obesity epidemic is a worldwide phenomenon. Nutr Rev 1998;56:106–14.
3. NAoS IoM. Nutrition in pregnancy. Part I. Weight gain. Part II nutrient supplements. Washington, DC: National Academies Press; 1990.
4. Yu CK, Teoh TG, Robinson S. Obesity in pregnancy. Br J Obstet Gynecol 2006;113:1117–25.
5. Heliovaara M, Aromaa A. Parity and obesity. J Epidemiol Community Health 1981;35:197–9.
6. Paladini D. Sonography in obese and overweight pregnant women: clinical, medicolegal and technical issues. Ultrasound Obstet Gynecol 2009;33: 720–9.
7. Bromley B, Shipp TD, Mitchell MA, et al. Tricks for obtaining a nuchal translucency measurement on the fetus in a difficult position. J Ultrasound Med 2010;29:1261–4.
8. Thornburg LL. Antepartum obstetrical complications associated with obesity. Semin Perinatol 2011;35: 317–23.
9. Magnavita N, Bevilacqua L, Mirk P, et al. Work-related musculoskeletal complaints in sonologists. J Occup Environ Med 1999;41:981–8.

10. Schoenfeld A, Goverman J, Weiss DM, et al. Transducer user syndrome: an occupational hazard of the ultrasonographer. Eur J Ultrasound 1999;10:41–5.
11. Paladini D, Vassallo M, Tartaglione A, et al. The role of tissue harmonic imaging in fetal echocardiography. Ultrasound Obstet Gynecol 2004;23:159–64.
12. Dashe JS, McIntire DD, Twickler DM. Effect of maternal obesity on the ultrasound detection of anomalous fetuses. Obstet Gynecol 2009;113:1001–7.
13. Malone FD, Canick JA, Ball RH, et al. First-trimester or second-trimester screening, or both, for Down's syndrome. N Engl J Med 2005;353:2001–11.
14. Wax JR, Pinette MG, Cartin A, et al. The value of repeated evaluation after initial failed nuchal translucency measurement. J Ultrasound Med 2007;26:825–8 [quiz: 29–30].
15. Thornburg LL, Mulconry M, Post A, et al. Fetal nuchal translucency thickness evaluation in the overweight and obese gravida. Ultrasound Obstet Gynecol 2009;33:665–9.
16. Gandhi M, Fox NS, Russo-Stieglitz K, et al. Effect of increased body mass index on first-trimester ultrasound examination for aneuploidy risk assessment. Obstet Gynecol 2009;114:856–9.
17. Tsai LJ, Ho M, Pressman EK, et al. Ultrasound screening for fetal aneuploidy using soft markers in the overweight and obese gravida. Prenat Diagn 2010;30:821–6.
18. Aagaard-Tillery KM, Flint Porter T, Malone FD, et al. Influence of maternal BMI on genetic sonography in the FaSTER trial. Prenat Diagn 2010;30:14–22.
19. Hendricks KA, Nuno OM, Suarez L, et al. Effects of hyperinsulinemia and obesity on risk of neural tube defects among Mexican Americans. Epidemiology 2001;12:630–5.
20. Waller DK, Mills JL, Simpson JL, et al. Are obese women at higher risk for producing malformed offspring? Am J Obstet Gynecol 1994;170:541–8.
21. Watkins ML, Rasmussen SA, Honein MA, et al. Maternal obesity and risk for birth defects. Pediatrics 2003;111:1152–8.
22. Waller DK, Shaw GM, Rasmussen SA, et al. Prepregnancy obesity as a risk factor for structural birth defects. Arch Pediatr Adolesc Med 2007;161:745–50.
23. Shaw GM, Velie EM, Schaffer D. Risk of neural tube defect-affected pregnancies among obese women. JAMA 1996;275:1093–6.
24. Watkins ML, Scanlon KS, Mulinare J, et al. Is maternal obesity a risk factor for anencephaly and spina bifida? Epidemiology 1996;7:507–12.
25. Queisser-Luft A, Kieninger-Baum D, Menger H, et al. Does maternal obesity increase the risk of fetal abnormalities? analysis of 20,248 newborn infants of the Mainz Birth Register for detecting congenital abnormalities. Ultraschall Med 1998;19:40–4 [in German].
26. Chung JH, Pelayo R, Hatfield TJ, et al. Limitations of the fetal anatomic survey via ultrasound in the obese obstetrical population. J Matern Fetal Neonatal Med 2012;25(10):1945–9.
27. Dashe JS, McIntire DD, Twickler DM. Maternal obesity limits the ultrasound evaluation of fetal anatomy. J Ultrasound Med 2009;28:1025–30.
28. Hendler I, Blackwell SC, Bujold E, et al. Suboptimal second-trimester ultrasonographic visualization of the fetal heart in obese women: should we repeat the examination? J Ultrasound Med 2005;24:1205–9 [quiz: 10–11].
29. Thornburg LL, Miles K, Ho M, et al. Fetal anatomic evaluation in the overweight and obese gravida. Ultrasound Obstet Gynecol 2009;33:670–5.
30. Maxwell C, Dunn E, Tomlinson G, et al. How does maternal obesity affect the routine fetal anatomic ultrasound? J Matern Fetal Neonatal Med 2010;23:1187–92.
31. Hendler I, Blackwell SC, Bujold E, et al. The impact of maternal obesity on midtrimester sonographic visualization of fetal cardiac and craniospinal structures. Int J Obes Relat Metab Disord 2004;28:1607–11.
32. Khoury FR, Ehrenberg HM, Mercer BM. The impact of maternal obesity on satisfactory detailed anatomic ultrasound image acquisition. J Matern Fetal Neonatal Med 2009;22:337–41.
33. Hendler I, Blackwell SC, Treadwell MC, et al. Does advanced ultrasound equipment improve the adequacy of ultrasound visualization of fetal cardiac structures in the obese gravid woman? Am J Obstet Gynecol 2004;190:1616–9 [discussion: 19–20].
34. Lantz ME, Chisholm CA. The preferred timing of second-trimester obstetric sonography based on maternal body mass index. J Ultrasound Med 2004;23:1019–22.
35. Jolly MC, Sebire NJ, Harris JP, et al. Risk factors for macrosomia and its clinical consequences: a study of 350,311 pregnancies. Eur J Obstet Gynecol Reprod Biol 2003;111:9–14.
36. Pressman EK, Bienstock JL, Blakemore KJ, et al. Prediction of birth weight by ultrasound in the third trimester. Obstet Gynecol 2000;95:502–6.
37. Alsulyman OM, Ouzounian JG, Kjos SL. The accuracy of intrapartum ultrasonographic fetal weight estimation in diabetic pregnancies. Am J Obstet Gynecol 1997;177:503–6.
38. Thornburg LL, Barnes C, Glantz JC, et al. Sonographic birth-weight prediction in obese patients using the gestation-adjusted prediction method. Ultrasound Obstet Gynecol 2008;32:66–70.
39. Best G, Pressman EK. Ultrasonographic prediction of birth weight in diabetic pregnancies. Obstet Gynecol 2002;99:740–4.

Ultrasonography for Fetal Lung Masses

Paula Zozzaro-Smith, DO

KEYWORDS

- Fetal lung lesions • Congenital cystic adenomatoid malformation
- Bronchopulmonary sequestration • Congenital high airway obstruction • Laryngeal atresia
- Bronchogenic cyst • Neurenteric cysts • Congenital lobar inflation

KEY POINTS

- Congenital cystic adenomatoid malformation (CCAM) is the most common congenital lung lesion, and results from a developmental abnormality of the respiratory tract.
- Bronchopulmonary sequestration (BPS) is a rare nonfunctional mass of lung tissue that does not communicate with the tracheobronchial tree and receives its arterial blood supply from the systemic vasculature rather than the pulmonary circulation.
- Hydrops fetalis can be a complication of both CCAM and BPS.
- A CCAM volume ratio (CVR) of 1.6 or greater predicts the development of hydrops.
- Pregnancies should be followed with serial ultrasonographic examinations to assess change in size of the lung mass, change in CVR, and development of hydrops.
- The presence of hydrops is a sign of impending fetal demise and is an indication for fetal intervention.
- Delivery should occur at a tertiary care facility with an intensive care nursery and staff, experienced in the resuscitation of a neonate with respiratory difficulties.

INTRODUCTION

The differential diagnosis of congenital lung masses includes a variety of lesions, with congenital cystic adenomatoid malformation (CCAM) and bronchopulmonary sequestration (BPS) being the most commonly encountered. The advent of prenatal ultrasonography has allowed for the increased identification of these lesions in addition to enhancing our knowledge regarding the natural history and potential clinical outcome of these lesions. This article serves to describe the diagnostic findings, prenatal management, and outcome of the most common fetal lung masses.

CONGENITAL CYSTIC ADENOMATOID MALFORMATION

CCAM, although rare, is the most common congenital lung lesion, and results from abnormal development of the lower respiratory tract.[1] In a majority of cases these lesions are usually unilateral involving a single lobe, although bilateral involvement can occur.[2] It can be distinguished from another fetal lung lesion, BPS, in that its blood supply originates from the existing pulmonary circulation.

CCAMs are presently classified into 5 types (0, 1, 2, 3, and 4) based on their histopathologic features including the size of the cysts and cellular characteristics. Type 0 is the rarest form, with involvement of the entire lung with resultant neonatal lethality caused by severe impairment of gas exchange. Type 1, characterized by large cysts 2 to 10 cm in diameter, is the most common form, comprising approximately 50% of CCAMs.[3] This type of CCAM has the potential for malignancy; however, the degree of risk has not been well defined.[4] Type 2 lesions typically are composed of smaller

Disclosures: None.
Division of Maternal Fetal Medicine, Department of Obstetrics and Gynecology, University of Rochester, 601 Elmwood Avenue, Box 668, Rochester, NY 14642, USA
E-mail address: Paula_Zozzaro-smith@URMC.rochester.edu

Ultrasound Clin 8 (2013) 49–54
http://dx.doi.org/10.1016/j.cult.2012.08.014
1556-858X/13/$ – see front matter

cysts and can be associated with other congenital anomalies in 60% of cases. These lesions include renal, other pulmonary, and cardiovascular anomalies. This type of lesion does not have malignant potential.[4] Type 3 CCAMs tend to be very large and can involve several lobes or the entire lung. These lesions are not associated with malignancy; however, type 4 lesions are composed of thick-walled cysts lined with alveolar lining cells and are strongly associated with malignancy, especially with pleuropulmonary blastoma.[4] This classification scheme is useful in the neonatal period; however, it has limited utility prenatally because tissue is not available for histologic examination.

Prenatal classification is based on ultrasonographic appearance, and classified as macrocystic or microcystic CCAMs. Macrocystic CCAMs typically have 1 or more cysts greater than 5 mm in size and are usually surrounded by hyperechogenic lung parenchyma (**Fig. 1**).[5] Lesions classified as microcystic appear as a solid hyperechogenic homogeneous mass compared with the surrounding lung parenchyma, secondary to the presence of cysts smaller than 5 mm (**Fig. 2**).[5] The arterial supply and venous drainage is primarily derived from the pulmonary circulation, although there may also be systemic connections present.[6] Contralateral mediastinal shift can occur with large lesions, with resultant compression of the inferior vena cava and heart, which can lead to hydrops fetalis (defined as 2 or more of the following: pleural effusion, pericardial effusion, skin edema, ascites, polyhydramnios) (**Figs. 3** and **4**). The esophagus can also become compressed and obstructed, resulting in polyhydramnios.

CCAMs can display a variable presentation ranging from incidental findings of cystic-appearing lesions to extensive pulmonary involvement. Lesions tend to regress throughout the course of gestation in as many as 50% of cases,

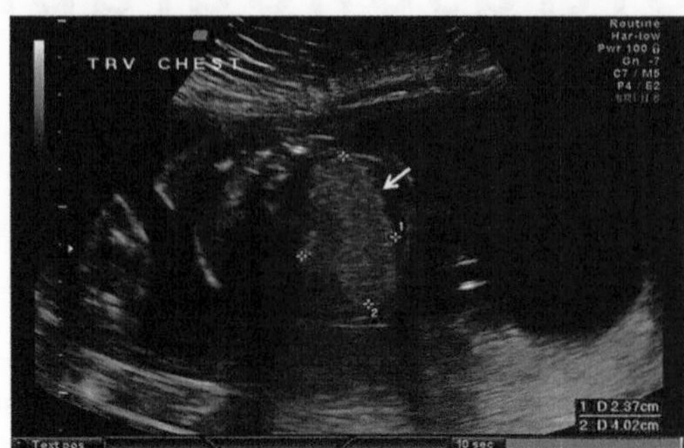

Fig. 2. Microcystic CCAM (*arrow*) visible on transverse view of fetal chest.

with peak CCAM size occurring at approximately 25 weeks gestational age.[7] However, fetal hydrops can develop in up to 40% of cases.[8] It is challenging to predict whether these masses will regress or grow and lead to hydrops. Certain mass features such as the appearance and the volume of the CCAM may be helpful in predicting complications. The volume of the CCAM adjusted for the gestational age may be a predictor for hydrops risk. A CCAM volume ratio (CVR) is obtained by dividing the congenital cystic adenomatoid malformation volume by head circumference to correct for fetal size. A CVR of greater than 1.6 is predictive of an increased risk of hydrops, with approximately 80% of these fetuses developing hydrops.[8] Despite obtaining a CVR, there are no reliable criteria for predicting which lesions will grow and result in hydrops. However, the presence of hydrops is the most important predictor of poor fetal outcome and is a sign of imminent fetal demise, with the risk of perinatal death approaching 100% without intervention.

Prenatal diagnosis is usually made by routine ultrasonography; however, prenatal magnetic resonance (MR) imaging may be useful in helping

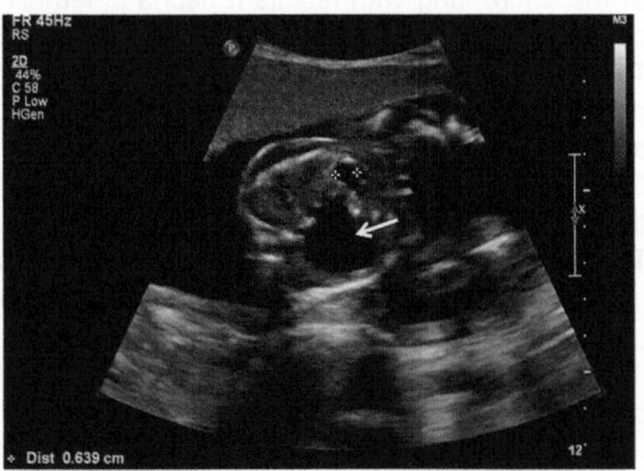

Fig. 1. Transverse view of fetal macrocystic CCAM (*arrow*).

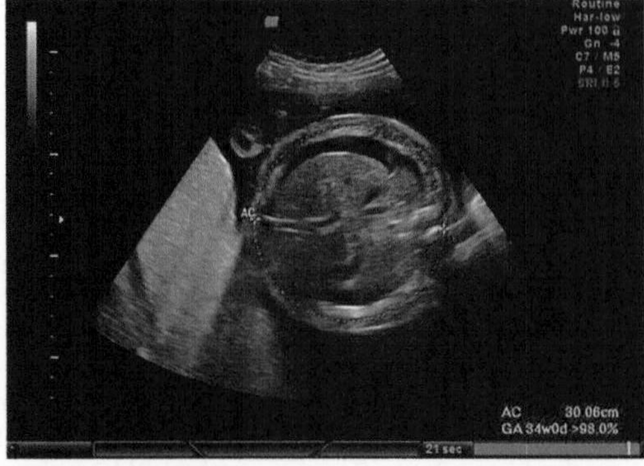

Fig. 3. Transverse image of abdominal ascites in a fetus with hydrops.

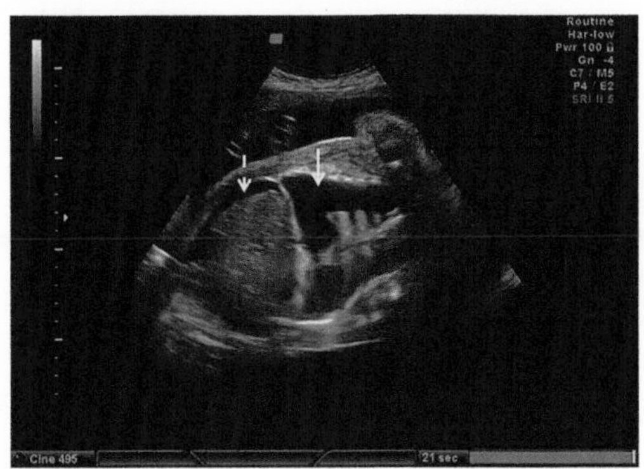

Fig. 4. Bilateral pleural effusions (*solid arrow*) and abdominal ascites (*dashed arrow*) in fetus with hydrops.

to distinguish CCAM from other less common lesions such as congenital diaphragmatic hernia. In one series, 90% of patients with fetal lung masses were diagnosed as CCAM by ultrasonography. However, MR imaging confirmed 60% of these lesions to be a CCAM, with the remainder being diagnosed as a congenital diaphragmatic hernia, BPS, or other less common lung lesions.[9] Another study also demonstrated the difficulty of prenatal sonographic diagnosis of CCAM with confirmation of 6 of 11 prenatally diagnosed cases of CCAM on final autopsy histopathology.[10] Hybrid lesions with histologic features of both CCAM and BPS have also been reported. These findings serve as a reminder that a prenatal diagnosis of CCAM by ultrasonography should not be considered conclusive.

Once a lung mass is noted, all patients should have serial prenatal follow-up ultrasonographic evaluations every 1 to 4 weeks to assess changes in size of the mass, CVR, and development of any additional complications including hydrops. The frequency of follow-up will depend on the size and CVR, with closer follow-up performed in those patients with a greater risk of developing hydrops. It is also important to perform a detailed ultrasound scan to evaluate for other congenital abnormalities. Other structural anomalies can be seen in approximately 10% of infants with CCAM, and can involve congenital anomalies of the gastrointestinal tract, bony anomalies, renal anomalies, and cardiac and central nervous system abnormalities.[11] Although isolated CCAMs typically are not associated with chromosomal abnormalities, in patients with additional ultrasonographic findings the risk of chromosomal abnormalities is increased and a fetal karyotype may be indicated.[12]

The presence of hydrops is an indication for fetal intervention. Without intervention, most fetuses with CCAMs and hydrops die in utero or shortly after delivery. For fetuses with hydrops at greater than 32 to 34 weeks gestational age, early delivery may be reasonable with postnatal resection. Before 32 weeks' gestation, several interventions to improve hydrops and prevent lung hypoplasia have been described.

Antenatal corticosteroids have been investigated as a potential medical intervention for CCAM. Their value was discovered when maternal betamethasone administration, 12 mg intramuscularly 2 doses 24 hours apart in anticipation of early delivery, appeared to reverse hydrops. In several uncontrolled studies with fetuses with predominantly microcystic CCAMs and a CVR of more than 1.6, hydrops resolved with prenatal steroid administration in approximately 80% of patients, with a majority surviving to delivery.[13,14] However, it must be noted that other studies have demonstrated resolution of hydrops without steroid administration, suggesting that possibly fetal growth and/or spontaneous regression of the lesion may have been responsible for hydrops resolution.[15,16]

Drainage procedures such as thoracentesis can be used to drain large pleural effusions to prevent pulmonary hypoplasia. Those lesions with a large macrocyst can also be aspirated to improve mediastinal shift. These strategies are mostly temporizing procedures, and fluid is likely to reaccumulate.[17] Thoracoamniotic shunting can be performed in utero to allow for cyst decompression; however, shunt placement can have technical limitations including displacement or catheter malfunction.[17] For CCAMs with a large solid component and hydrops before 32 weeks' gestation, in utero open resection has been successfully performed with resolution of the hydrops over a few weeks. In one series, surgical resection was performed in fetuses at 21 to 29 weeks' gestation, with 60% of survivors displaying resolution of hydrops and improvement in lung growth.[18]

A lung mass that is small in size with no mediastinal shift or hydrops is not an indication for early delivery or cesarean delivery. Delivery should occur at a tertiary care facility with an intensive care nursery and staff experienced in the resuscitation of a neonate with respiratory difficulties.

Postnatally, CCAM is often treated by surgical resection in an effort to treat significant respiratory distress, or electively to prevent recurrent infection and to eliminate concerns regarding malignancy. The timing of elective resection is controversial with the optimal age for surgery suggested as between 3 and 6 months of age. Alternatively, observation with serial chest computed tomographic imaging can be another approach to surgical resection. The disadvantages of this approach are the risk of malignant transformation, infection, and radiation exposure.

BRONCHOPULMONARY SEQUESTRATION

A BPS is a rare nonfunctional mass of lung tissue that does not communicate with the tracheobronchial tree and receives its arterial blood supply from the systemic vasculature rather than the pulmonary circulation. Most commonly, the feeder vessel originates from the aorta; however, vessels from the gastric and the splenic artery as well as multiple feeding vessels have been described.[19] The embryologic etiology of BPS is unclear, but is believed to occur early in embryonic development before the division of the aortic and pulmonary circulations.

Sequestrations are classified into 2 forms based on their location: intralobar, in which the lesion is surrounded by normal lung tissue, and extralobar, in which the mass is located outside the normal lung and is completely enclosed in its own pleura.[8] Postnatally, intralobar sequestration is overall the most common type, accounting for approximately 80% of sequestrations, and most have no bronchial connection to the proximal airway.[20] These lesions may have abnormal connections to other bronchi and the gastrointestinal tract, which may allow bacteria to enter and result in recurrent infection. Extralobar sequestrations also lack a bronchial connection; however, they also may connect to the gastrointestinal tract or, rarely, to intrapulmonary structures.

Most cases are identified by routine prenatal ultrasonography, and diagnosis is suggested by the presence of a solid echogenic triangular mass with an occasional cystic component often seen in the lower chest near the diaphragm (**Fig. 5**).[21] Lesions are usually unilateral, although bilateral cases have been described.[22] These sequestrations are distinguished from CCAMs based on identification of a systemic artery to the lung lesion by color flow Doppler (**Fig. 6**).[23] Mediastinal shift is often seen. Prenatal MR imaging may also be helpful in distinguishing sequestrations from other common lung lesions.

In most cases, the lesion will likely decrease in size; however, the potential for hydrops still may exist as a result of vascular compression.[8] There are no reliable criteria for determining which lesions will grow and develop hydrops. All patients should have serial prenatal follow-up ultrasound scans to assess changes in size as well as development of hydrops. When identified, a thorough assessment should be performed to assess for additional anomalies. Other congenital anomalies such as congenital diaphragmatic hernia, vertebral

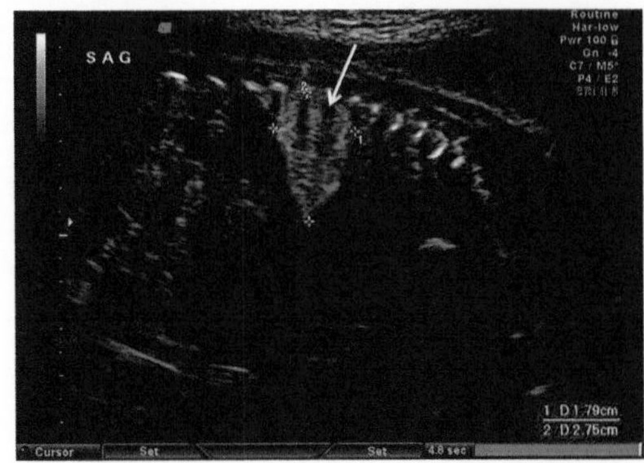

Fig. 5. Sagittal view of fetal bronchopulmonary sequestration (*arrow*).

anomalies, and congenital heart disease may be seen with BPS, most frequently in patients with an extralobar sequestration.[24] The incidence of chromosomal abnormalities is not increased with BPS alone; however, this risk is increased with additional anomalies.

Most sequestrations regress or completely disappear during prenatal life. Few develop hydrops and thus fetal intervention is rarely needed, and fetuses do well with surgical removal after birth. If the fetus develops pleural effusions or a macrocyst is present as a result of a hybrid lesion, thoracentesis or thoracoamniotic shunting may be used. A lung mass that is small in size with no mediastinal shift or hydrops is not an indication for early delivery or cesarean delivery. Delivery should occur at a tertiary care facility with an intensive care nursery and staff experienced in the resuscitation of a neonate with respiratory difficulties.

Postnatally, the most common complication of BPS is pulmonary infection.[24] Rare complications can include heart failure caused by increased flow through the feeding artery and massive hemorrhage.[25] BPS is treated by surgical excision

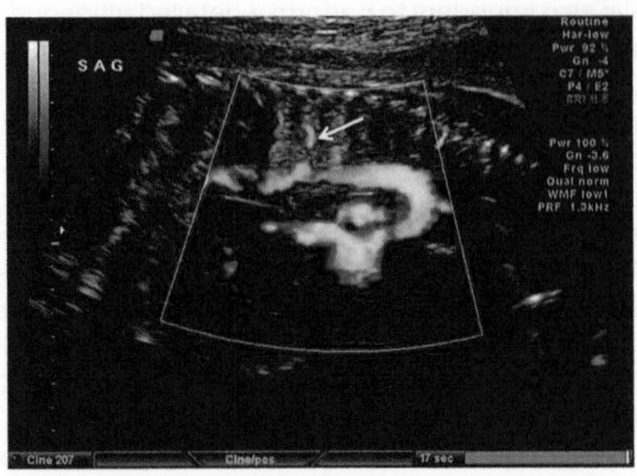

Fig. 6. Systemic feeder vessel arising from aorta to sequestration (*arrow*).

both for symptoms and to prevent infection, with ligation of all vascular connections to the lesion.[24]

CONGENITAL HIGH AIRWAY OBSTRUCTION (LARYNGEAL ATRESIA)

Congenital high airway obstruction results from obstruction of the upper airway, most commonly as a result of laryngeal atresia. It is diagnosed by prenatal ultrasonography by the findings of large hyperechogenic lungs, flattened or inverted diaphragms, dilated distal airways, and fetal hydrops (**Fig. 7**). Obstruction leads to impairment of flow of lung fluid, with distension of the tracheobronchial tree and lung expansion leading to tracheobronchomalacia and respiratory distress syndrome. The enlarged lungs cause cardiovascular compression and heart failure with resultant ascites and hydrops.[26]

Current knowledge regarding the natural history of congenital high airway obstruction is limited because of its rarity. Based on the limited cases described it has been considered lethal; however, the prognosis may be more favorable if a fistula through the obstructed airway is present to allow for the release of intrathoracic pressure. If diagnosed antenatally, intensive care immediately following delivery is necessary, which includes an emergent tracheostomy. Surgical correction is possible, but the prognosis for survival remains poor. Ex utero intrapartum treatment (EXIT) has marginally improved the prognosis of those fetuses diagnosed prenatally with laryngeal atresia, with a limited number of case reports describing successful management.[27]

OTHER LUNG ABNORMALITIES

Other rarer lung lesions include congenital lobar inflation, bronchogenic cysts, and neurenteric

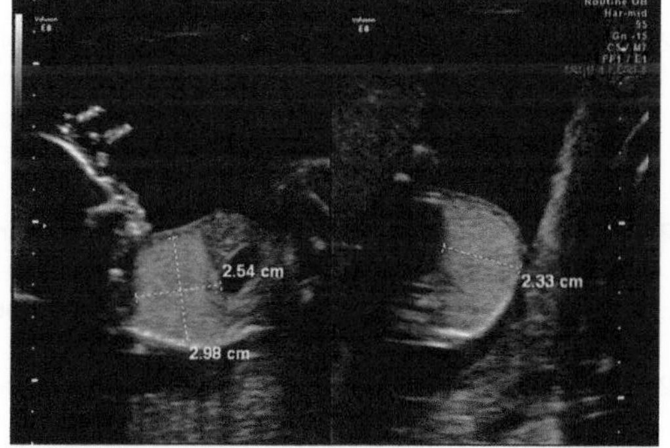

Fig. 7. Prenatal ultrasound scan demonstrating a fetal lung mass involving entire left chest, consistent with congenital high airway obstruction on fetal magnetic resonance imaging.

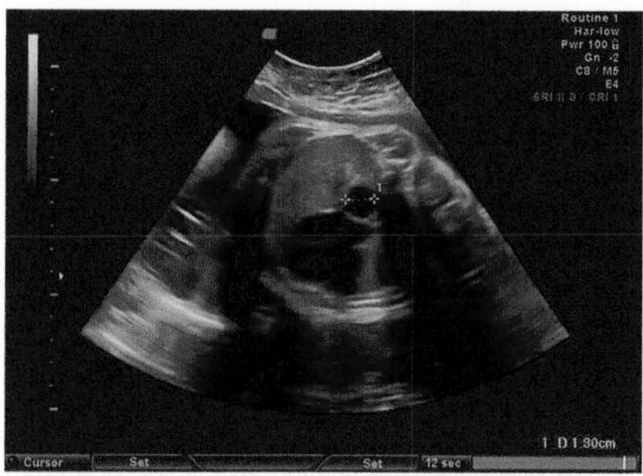

Fig. 8. Simple cystic lung lesion on transverse fetal chest consistent with bronchogenic cyst on final histopathology.

cysts. Congenital lobar inflation results from obstruction of segment or lobe of the lung that results in progressive hyperexpansion of the lung parenchyma. A prenatal diagnosis is uncommon, but has been described as an echogenic mass with associated compression of the remaining lung.[28]

Bronchogenic cysts are caused by the abnormal ventral budding of the tracheobronchial tree, which results in a focal cystic duplication. These cysts typically present as a single fluid filled cyst varying in size from a few millimeters to greater than 5 cm (**Fig. 8**). Less commonly, they may present as multiple lesions.[29]

Neurenteric cysts result from incomplete separation of the notochord from the foregut in the third to fourth weeks of embryonic development. The majority are located in the right posterior mediastinum, with associated vertebral anomalies present in about 50% of these lesions. The cysts may be unilocular with internal septations. Potentially they can displace and compress adjacent structures such as the lungs, heart, and vessels, as well as cause central nervous system symptoms with intraspinal lesions.[30]

SUMMARY

Congenital lung lesions comprise a spectrum of developmental anomalies and causes, with the most common being CCAM and BPS. With the advent of prenatal ultrasonography, our understanding and evaluation of these lesions have improved alongside an increase in antenatal detection. Although the majority of anomalies of the fetal lungs can be visualized on routine ultrasonography, this modality has a low specificity whereby a definitive diagnosis is usually only accomplished on surgical resection and histopathologic evaluation. Therefore, patients presenting with a fetal lung mass should undergo a thorough ultrasonographic examination to exclude other congenital abnormalities, and be followed serially with further sonographic evaluations to assess progression in size and the development of potential lethal complications such as hydrops.

REFERENCES

1. Calvert JK, Lakhoo K. Antenatally suspected congenital cystic adenomatoid malformation of the lung: postnatal investigation and timing of surgery. J Pediatr Surg 2007;42:411–4.
2. Adzick NS. Management of fetal lung lesions. Clin Perinatol 2009;36:363–76.
3. Laje P, Liechty KW. Postnatal management and outcome of prenatally diagnosed lung lesions. Prenat Diagn 2008;28:612–8.
4. Priest JR, Williams GM, Hill DA, et al. Pulmonary cysts in early childhood and the risk of malignancy. Pediatr Pulmonol 2009;44:14–30.
5. Adzick NS. Management of fetal lung lesions. Clin Perinatol 2003;30:481–92.
6. Tsao K, Albanese CT, Harrison MR. Prenatal therapy for thoracic and mediastinal lesions. World J Surg 2003;27:77–83.
7. Laberge JM, Flageole H, Pugash D, et al. Outcome of the prenatally diagnosed congenital cystic adenomatoid lung malformation: a Canadian experience. Fetal Diagn Ther 2001;16(3):178–86.
8. Azizkhan RG, Crombleholme TM. Congenital cystic lung disease: contemporary antenatal and postnatal management. Pediatr Surg Int 2008;24:643–57.
9. Hubbard AM, Adzick NS, Crombleholme TM, et al. Congenital chest lesions: diagnosis and characterization with prenatal MR imaging. Radiology 1999; 212(1):43–8.
10. Harmath A, Csaba A, Hauzman E, et al. Congenital lung malformations in the second trimester: prenatal ultrasound diagnosis and pathologic findings. J Clin Ultrasound 2007;35(5):250–5.
11. Schott S, Mackensen-Haen S, Wallwiener M, et al. Cystic adenomatoid malformation of the lung causing hydrops fetalis: case report and review of the literature. Arch Gynecol Obstet 2009;280:293–6.
12. Bush A, Hogg J, Chitty L. Cystic lung lesions—prenatal diagnosis and management. Prenat Diagn 2008;28:604–11.
13. Curran PF, Jelin EB, Rand L, et al. Prenatal steroids for microcystic congenital cystic adenomatoid malformations. J Pediatr Surg 2010;45:145–50.
14. Peranteau WH, Wilson RD, Liechty KW, et al. Effect of maternal betamethasone administration on prenatal congenital cystic adenomatoid malformation growth and fetal survival. Fetal Diagn Ther 2007;22(5):365–71.
15. Crombleholme TM, Coleman B, Hedrick H, et al. Cystic adenomatoid malformation volume ratio predicts outcome in prenatally diagnosed cystic adenomatoid malformation of the lung. J Pediatr Surg 2002;37:331–7.
16. Kunisaki SM, Barnewolt CE, Estroff JA, et al. Large fetal congenital cystic adenomatoid malformations: growth trends and patient survival. J Pediatr Surg 2007;42:404–10.
17. Mann S, Wilson RD, Bebbington MW, et al. Antenatal diagnosis and management of congenital cystic adenomatoid malformation. Semin Fetal Neonatal Med 2007;12:477–81.
18. Adzick NS, Harrison MR, Crombleholme TM, et al. Fetal lung lesions: management and outcome. Am J Obstet Gynecol 1998;179(4):884–9.
19. Gomez L, Robert JA, Sepulveda W. Fetal retroperitoneal pulmonary sequestration with an atypical vascular pattern. Prenat Diagn 2009;29:290–1.
20. Abbey P, Das CJ, Pangtey GS, et al. Imaging in bronchopulmonary sequestration. J Med Imaging Radiat Oncol 2009;53:22–31.
21. Sepulveda W. Perinatal imaging in bronchopulmonary sequestration. J Ultrasound Med 2009;28:89–94.
22. Stern R, Berger S, Casaulta C, et al. Bilateral intralobar pulmonary sequestration in a newborn, case report and review of the literature on bilateral pulmonary sequestrations. J Pediatr Surg 2007;42:E19–23.
23. Vijayaraghavan SB, Rao PS, Selvarasu CD, et al. Prenatal sonographic features of intralobar bronchopulmonary sequestration. J Ultrasound Med 2003; 22:541–4.
24. Gezer S, Tastepe I, Sirmali M, et al. Pulmonary sequestration: a single-institutional series composed of 27 cases. J Thorac Cardiovasc Surg 2007;133:955–9.
25. Levine MM, Nudel DB, Gootman N, et al. Pulmonary sequestration causing congestive heart failure in infancy: a report of two cases and review of the literature. Ann Thorac Surg 1982;34:581.
26. Hamid-Sowinka A, Ropacka-Lesiak M, Breborowicz GH. Congenital high airway obstruction syndrome. Neuro Endocrinol Lett 2011;32(5):623–6.
27. Kanamori Y, Kitano Y, Hashizume K, et al. A case of laryngeal atresia (congenital high airway obstruction syndrome) with chromosome 5p deletion syndrome rescued by ex utero intrapartum treatment. J Pediatr Surg 2004;39(1):E25.
28. Quinton AE, Smoleniec JS. Congenital lobar emphysema-the disappearing chest mass: antenatal ultrasound appearance. Ultrasound Obstet Gynecol 2001;17:169–71.
29. Correia-Pinto J, Gonzaga S, Huang Y, et al. Congenital lung lesions—underlying molecular mechanisms. Semin Pediatr Surg 2010;19:171–9.
30. Macaulay KE, Winter TC, Shields LE. Neurenteric cyst shown by prenatal sonography. Am J Roentgenol 1997;169(2):563–5.

Ultrasound for Abdominal Wall Defects

Elizabeth A. Fountaine, MD[a],
Kristin M. Knight, MD, FACOG[b,*]

KEYWORDS

• Abdominal wall defect • Congenital anomaly • Gastroschisis • Omphalocele

KEY POINTS

- Abdominal wall defects are common congenital malformations affecting 1 in 2,000 live births.
- Accurate prenatal diagnosis of the type of abdominal wall defect is important for determining prognosis and optimizing fetal/neonatal outcome.
- Various abdominal wall defects can be distinguished prenatally based on a number of sonographic characteristics.

 **Videos of a second-trimester fetus with gastroschisis accompany this article.**

OVERVIEW AND CLINICAL SIGNIFICANCE

Fetal abdominal wall defects occur in 1 in 2,000 live births. Prevalent use of antenatal ultrasonography and maternal serum α-fetoprotein screening has led to increasing detection of abdominal wall defects. In fact, owing to increased use of first trimester ultrasound, a majority of fetal abdominal wall defects are now detected as early as 11 to 14 weeks of gestation. In essence, ultrasound by 12 weeks of gestation should be able to detect all cases of omphalocele and gastroschisis (the 2 most common abdominal wall defects).[1,2] **Table 1** describes the most common types of abdominal wall defects.

EMBRYOLOGIC DEVELOPMENT OF THE ABDOMINAL WALL

During the 4th and 5th weeks of development, the flat embryonic disk folds in 4 directions: Cephalic, caudal, left lateral, and right lateral (**Table 2**). The folds converge at the site of the umbilicus and therefore obliterate the extra-embryonic coelom. During this period of fetal development, the liver and bowel are also rapidly growing.[3,4]

During the 6th week of fetal development, abdominal cavity growth lags behind the growth of internal structures, mainly the bowel. This temporary disproportionate growth causes a physiologic protrusion of the intestines into the residual extra-embryonic coelom at the location of the umbilical cord insertion, termed the physiologic midgut herniation. This process can be appreciated ultrasonographically between 9 and 11 weeks of gestation. If this herniation is appreciated beyond 12 weeks, it is no longer considered physiologic.[5]

GASTROSCHISIS

Gastroschisis occurs when fetal intestines eviscerate through a full-thickness abdominal wall defect. The defect is paraumbilical, most commonly occurring to the right of the umbilicus. The

Disclosures: The authors report no conflicts of interest.

[a] Department of Obstetrics and Gynecology, University of Rochester, 601 Elmwood Avenue, Box 668, Rochester, NY 14642, USA; [b] Maternal-Fetal Medicine Associates of Maryland, 10110 Molecular Drive, Suite #218, Rockville, MD 20850
* Corresponding author.
E-mail address: kristinmaeknight@gmail.com

Ultrasound Clin 8 (2013) 55–67
http://dx.doi.org/10.1016/j.cult.2012.08.016

Table 1
Epidemiology of the most common types of abdominal wall defects

Type of Abdominal Wall Defect	Incidence (Live Births)	Epidemiology
Gastroschisis	1/4,000	Most cases sporadic 1:1 ratio of male: female ↑ incidence in young mothers (<20) ↑ incidence of maternal smoking ↑ incidence in Caucasians ↑ incidence in 1st-born fetuses
Omphalocele	1/4,000	Most cases sporadic 40% with chromosomal anomaly ↑ at extremes of reproductive age (↑chromosomal link if liver intracorporeal)
Ectopia cordis/pentalogy of Cantrell	<1/100,000 (Only ~90 reported cases of complete pentalogy syndrome – most partial)	Most cases sporadic 2:1 ratio of male:female Most cases involve incomplete forms of the syndrome
Limb–body wall complex/body stalk	0.3/100,000	Most cases sporadic 50% cases associated with maternal smoking 50% cases associated with maternal alcohol use 40% had prior infant with congenital anomaly
Cloacal exstrophy	1/200,000	Most cases sporadic Genetics not well-defined, but ↑incidence in families with affected individual
Bladder exstrophy	1/30,000 (↑ to 1:70 in offspring of affected individuals)	Most cases sporadic 3:1 ratio of male: female Increased frequency in 1st born Increased frequency in Caucasians

Data from Refs.[2,33,57,58]

defect itself is not covered by any membrane, leaving the fetal bowel directly exposed to surrounding amniotic fluid. Embryologically, gastroschisis is thought to be caused by vascular occlusion of the omphalomesenteric or umbilical vein.[6–8] No studies have proven association with any chromosomal anomaly, including aneuploidy.

Table 2
Embryonic disc folds and corresponding abdominal quadrant

Disc Folds	Abdominal Quadrant
Cephalic fold	Epigastrium
Caudal fold	Hypogastrium
Right lateral fold	Right lateral abdominal wall
Left lateral fold	Left lateral abdominal wall

Data from Duhamel B. Embryology of exomphalos and allied malformations. Arch Dis Child 1963;38:142.

Clinically, the prevalence of chromosomal abnormalities in fetuses with isolated gastroschisis is not increased above baseline risk. Owing to an increased risk of intrauterine growth restriction and concern of loss of fluid and protein across the exposed bowel, it is recommended that increased antenatal surveillance is instituted at 30 to 32 weeks of gestation with twice-weekly nonstress testing or weekly assessment of the biophysical profile score.[9] Because of an increased risk of preterm delivery (although 70% of fetuses with gastroschisis deliver at ≥37 weeks of gestation) and subsequent neonatal complications, delivery at a tertiary care center is recommended.

A meta-analysis of observational studies evaluating the effect of mode of delivery on fetuses with abdominal wall defects (gastroschisis and omphalocele) concluded there was no relationship between mode of delivery and rate of primary fascial repair, neonatal sepsis, pediatric mortality, time until enteral feeding, or length of hospital stay.[10]

OMPHALOCELE

An omphalocele is a herniation of abdominal contents into a medial abdominal wall defect. This occurs most commonly at the base of the umbilical cord, with the cord insertion located at the apex of the herniated sac. The defect itself is covered by a membrane consisting of the amnion and peritoneum.[2,11]

Embryologically, a simple midline omphalocele develops when the extra-embryonic gut fails to return to the abdominal cavity and remains covered by the amniotic-peritoneal membrane. If the lateral folds fail to close and the subsequent abdominal wall defect is large enough, abdominal contents, including the liver, can herniate. If the liver is included in the external herniation, this condition is termed a liver-containing (or "giant") omphalocele.[3,4,12] There is typically no association of increased risk of aneuploidy with liver-containing omphaloceles; therefore, karyotype testing is not routinely performed.

Non–liver-containing omphaloceles solely contain bowel. Owing to normal physiologic midgut herniation in the first trimester, an accurate diagnosis of true non–liver-containing omphalocele cannot be made reliably before 12 weeks of gestation.[5,13] Because of the strong association with aneuploidy in fetuses with this form of omphalocele, a karyotype is recommended during prenatal testing (**Table 3**).

Omphaloceles are often associated with other fetal anomalies, most commonly cardiac, genitourinary, and other gastrointestinal anomalies. Fetal growth restriction and neural tube defects are often seen as well.[14] The prevalence of omphalocele in the setting of increased nuchal translucency is increased 10-fold from baseline, even in the setting of normal chromosome testing.[15] Omphaloceles are also appreciated as a part of a constellation of features including macroglossia, visceromegaly, and neonatal hypoglycemia.[16] This unique combination of findings is found in the following disorders: Pentalogy of Cantrell, schisis association, omphalocele–exstrophy–imperforate anus–spinal defects syndrome, Beckwith-Wiedemann syndrome, and amniotic band syndrome. A subset of these disorders will be discussed below.

Clinically, 95% of omphaloceles are accurately diagnosed on ultrasound. Maternal serum α-fetoprotein concentration is elevated in 70% of cases. Workup with a fetal karyotype is useful to assess for a chromosomal abnormality. In addition, Beckwith-Wiedemann syndrome testing should be considered if indicated. Fetal echocardiograms are also recommended owing to the 50% incidence of congenital cardiac anomalies in infants with an omphalocele. As with gastroschisis, fetal growth restriction is common and antenatal surveillance with nonstress testing and/or ultrasound should begin at 30 to 32 weeks' gestation.[9]

CLOACAL EXSTROPHY

Cloacal exstrophy is a constellation of findings seen in infants who embryologically experienced abnormal folding of the ventral abdominal wall. It is considered the most severe of the exstrophy-epispadias complex disorders.[17] The spectrum

Table 3
Types of omphalocele

	Liver-Containing Omphalocele	Non–Liver-Containing Omphalocele
Gestational age at sonographic diagnosis	As early as 9–10 weeks by transvaginal ultrasound	A reliable diagnosis cannot be made until 12 weeks or later owing to physiologic midgut herniation before that gestational age
Association with aneuploidy	Rare	40% of fetuses
Sonographic appearance	A homogenous appearing mass measuring >5–10 mm in diameter within the midgut herniation consistent with liver	Echogenic material consistent with bowel protruding through midgut herniation after 12 weeks gestational age

Data from Refs.[2,13,33]

of disease includes some or all of the following findings: Hypogastric omphalocele, meningomyelocele, scoliosis, abnormal genitalia, kidneys, and female reproductive organs into an extracorporeal sac and/or herniation of the bladder.

Embryologically, cloacal exstrophy results from failure of mesodermal cell migration with subsequent abnormal caudal folding. Extensive failure of the caudal fold somatic layer leads to absence of the hypogastric wall in front of the allantois, thereby producing urorectal or cloacal exstrophy as well as omphalocele.[3]

Clinically, fetal karyotyping may be useful to detect a possible chromosomal abnormality; however, cloacal exstrophy itself has not been directly linked with any particular abnormality. In addition to aiding with prognosis, fetal karyotype determination may also be useful in terms of gender assignment postnatally, because it is often difficult to visually distinguish male from female genitalia in severe cases. Delivery at a tertiary care center is recommended. Vaginal delivery is preferred if possible, with cesarean delivery reserved for the usual obstetric indications. Care should be taken while ligating the umbilical cord to ensure that extra-abdominal viscera are excluded. Survival rates of 83% to 100% have been reported at tertiary care centers, although quality-of-life concerns remain an issue for many of these infants in adulthood.[18] Associated anomalies include anorectal atresia, abdominal wall defects, pelvic anomalies, and spinal column abnormalities.

BLADDER EXSTROPHY

Bladder exstrophy is a spectrum of anomalies of the bladder, inferior abdominal wall, external genitalia, and bony pelvis. It is considered a milder form of the exstrophy-epispadias complex compared with the more severe cloacal exstrophy. Mild cases of bladder exstrophy involve simple exstrophy of the urethra alone or in addition to a portion of the bladder. Severe cases involve separation of the symphysis pubis and often are accompanied by an abnormally positioned anal orifice.[19]

Embryologically, bladder exstrophy occurs owing to maldevelopment of the lower abdominal wall, resulting in failure to close during fetal development. The most universally accepted theory for the cause of abnormal lower abdominal wall development was proposed by Marshall and Muecke.[20] They postulate that development of the abdominal wall is disrupted by the overdevelopment of the cloacal membrane, thus preventing medial migration of the mesenchymal tissue toward the midline. The cloacal membrane eventually ruptures, resulting in protrusion of the anterior bladder wall through the lower abdominal wall. The bladder thus communicates with the surrounding amniotic fluid.

Clinically, these infants have an exposed bladder and posterior urethra. The umbilicus sits just above the defect, in a more caudal position than normal. The symphysis pubis also displays separation secondary to outward malrotation of the hip girdle. The perineum is shortened with the anus positioned more anteriorly than normal, forming the inferior boundary of the fascial defect. Male infants frequently experience epispadias and open prostate glands, which lie posterior to the urethra rather than encircling it.[21] Female infants often experience a bifid clitoris with epispadias and small, laterally displaced labia minora.[22]

LIMB–BODY WALL COMPLEX

Body stalk anomalies refer to a group of lethal malformations in which abdominal wall defects are so significant the abdominal, and often thoracic, organs lie outside the body cavity and within a membrane composed of amnion and peritoneum. This sac is most often directly attached to the placenta. The main features of this abnormality are large complex cranial defects (eg, encephalocele), facial clefts, body wall defects of the thorax and/or abdominal wall, and limb defects. The umbilical cord may be totally absent or extremely shortened. Severe kyphoscoliosis is often present.[23]

Embryologically, limb–body wall complex disorders occur from failure of fusion of all 4 embryonic disc folds during the 6th postmenstrual week. Normally, after the embryo folds, the intra-embryonic coelom (future peritoneal cavity) is separated from the extra-embryonic coelom, and the umbilical cord subsequently forms. If this folding does not occur, then the extra-embryonic cavity is not obliterated and the body stalk is missing.[24] Herniation of abdominal contents into the amnioperitoneal sac occurs owing to lack of lateral folding. Additionally, abnormal caudal folding results in the malformations noted with cloacal exstrophy. Severe scoliosis develops as a consequence of the irregular attachment of the fetus to the placenta.[25]

This syndrome is often detected by prenatal ultrasound in the second trimester. A combination of scoliosis and omphalocele should suggest this diagnosis, which has been made as early as the 9th postmenstrual week.[3] Criteria for first trimester ultrasound diagnosis include demonstration of the internal viscera in the extra-embryonic coelom and a short, 2-vessel umbilical cord.[26] Differential diagnosis includes amniotic band syndrome.

Associated abnormalities include craniofacial abnormalities (encephalocele, holocranium), mid-facial clefts, increased nuchal translucency,[27] limb defects, and significant skeletal abnormalities. Clinically, termination should be offered, because this abnormality is always lethal.

PENTALOGY OF CANTRELL

Pentalogy of Cantrell (or thoraco-abdominal syndrome) is a rare and complex malformation caused by failure of cephalic body folding. This syndrome is most often found in partial form; presence of complete Pentalogy is exceptionally rare. The disorder is characterized by the following features: Median supraumbilical abdominal defect, defect of the lower sternum (sternal cleft), deficiency of the diaphragmatic pericardium (ectopia cordis), deficiency of the anterior diaphragm (anterior diaphragmatic hernia), and intracardiac abnormalities.[28]

The diagnosis should be considered if both ectopia cordis and an omphalocele/ventral abdominal wall defect have been demonstrated. The intrathoracic abnormalities may be difficult to detect. Ectopia cordis itself is a rare defect in which the heart is partially or completely exposed on the surface of the thorax. Up to 80% of affected fetuses have associated intracardiac defects, including ventricular septal defects, tetralogy of Fallot, left ventricular diverticulum, double outlet right ventricle, and pulmonary hypoplasia.[29]

Embryologically, ectopia cordis results from failure of fusion of the lateral folds in the primitive fetal thorax during the 6th postmenstrual week. It is classified as 1 of 4 types: Cervical (3%), thoracic (60%), thoraco-abdominal (7%), and abdominal (30%).[30] Complete pentalogy of Cantrell has been postulated to occur secondary to an error of mesodermal migration occurring between days 14 and 18 of the embryonic period.

Clinically, this malformation has been detected as early as postmenstrual week 10 or 11. Antenatal 3-dimensional ultrasonography is useful to better characterize the anomaly. Neonatal mortality is very high, especially with complete thoracic ectopia cordis, which, if left untreated, is universally lethal.[31] Associated abnormalities include craniofacial defects, trisomies 18, 13, and 21, and cystic hygroma.

Clinically, survival is variable but uncommon. Prognosis ultimately depends on the size of the abdominal wall defect, the extent of the cardiac defect, and presence or absence of associated anomalies.

IMAGING PROTOCOLS

Sonographic evaluation of the fetal anterior abdominal wall, cord insertion, and bladder are part of the standard anatomic survey in the second and third trimesters.[32] If these structures are adequately visualized and normal in appearance, the vast majority of fetal abdominal wall defects are excluded. Common limitations precluding adequate visualization of the umbilical cord insertion into the abdominal wall are oligohydramnios and advanced gestational age; in these scenarios, the absence of an abdominal wall defect often cannot be confirmed.

If an abdominal wall defect is suspected, the following approach to evaluating the abnormality has been recommended[2]:

1. Evaluate for the presence of a limiting membrane;
2. Evaluate the relationship between the umbilical cord and the defect;
3. Identify the eviscerated organs;
4. Assess the bowel appearance; and
5. Evaluate for the presence of additional fetal malformations.

In clinical practice, this approach is highly useful in distinguishing between the various abdominal wall defects (**Table 4**).

IMAGING FINDINGS

Evaluation for the Presence of a Limiting Membrane

This initial step in the evaluation of a suspected abdominal wall defect will help to distinguish between the 2 most common defects, gastroschisis and omphalocele. With an omphalocele, the eviscerated abdominal contents will be contained within a membrane composed of peritoneum and amnion (**Fig. 1**).[2,11] This membrane is often visible; however, in some cases when there is limited visualization, the membrane may not be directly visualized and the eviscerated abdominal contents will seem to be contained, suggesting the presence of a membrane.[2] In the case of gastroschisis, the eviscerated abdominal contents are not contained within a membrane and are therefore freely floating in the amniotic cavity. Because the majority of cases of gastroschisis involve extra-abdominal small bowel, these cases often have a "cauliflower-like" appearance (**Figs. 2** and **3**).[11] Videos 1 and 2 are clips of scanning through the abdominal wall of a fetus with gastroschisis. One potential pitfall can occur when a large amount of fetal ascites is present. In this case, the eviscerated contents may appear free-floating; however, they are floating in ascites rather than amniotic fluid

Table 4
Sonographic characteristics of the most common abdominal wall defects

Type of Defect	Limiting Membrane	Umbilical Cord Insertion	Extracorporeal Organs	Appearance of Bowel	Associated Malformations
Gastroschisis	Absent	Paraumbilical defect	Small bowel	Dilated and thickened	Coexistent bowel defects (ischemia, malrotation, atresia) Growth restriction
Omphalocele	Present	Defect connected to cord insertion at apex of mass	Small bowel Liver can be intra-/extra-corporeal	Normal Ascites is common	Other fetal anomaly (70%) Chromosomal anomaly (40%) Cardiac defect (50%) Thick nuchal fold (↑10 fold) GI/GU anomalies Growth restriction
Limb–body complex	Present	Defect connected to cord insertion (umbilicus and true cord absent or shortened)	+/- heart +/- lungs +/- liver +/- spleen +/- kidneys +/- bladder +/- female reproductive organs	Abnormal (varies pending extent of deformity)	Craniofacial abnormalities Limb defects (95% cases) Midfacial clefts Scoliosis Thick nuchal fold (71%) ↑ MS α-fetoprotein (100% cases)
Bladder exstrophy	Absent	Defect below level of cord insertion	Bladder Dorsal urethra	Normal	Inguinal hernia (82% males, 15% female)
Cloacal exstrophy	Variable	Defect below level of cord insertion If omphalocele – defect connected to cord insertion	Bladder +/- kidneys +/- female reproductive organs	Hypoplasia of the colon is common	Anorectal atresia Abdominal wall defect (omphalocele) Renal/urinary anomaly (50%) Pelvic anomalies (30%) Spinal column abnormalities (meningomyelocele) Single Umbilical Artery
Pentalogy of Cantrell	Present	Defect above level of cord insertion	Heart	Normal	Craniofacial defects Trisomy 13, 18, 21 Cystic hygroma

Data from Refs.[2,27,59–62]

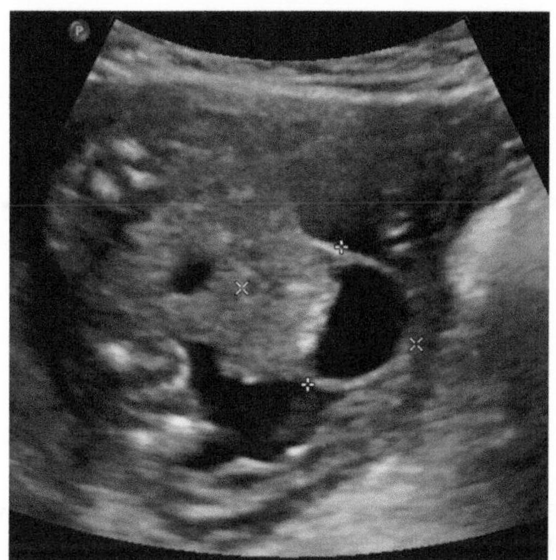

Fig. 1. Transverse abdominal view of a second-trimester fetus with an omphalocele. Note the clearly demarcated surrounding membrane. The calipers mark the boundaries of the extra-abdominal portion of the abdominal contents.

(**Fig. 4**).[2] Therefore, attempts should be made to identify the surrounding membrane when at all possible. An additional pitfall is the case of a ruptured omphalocele. Although a rare entity,[2] it has the potential of causing diagnostic confusion because the extra-abdominal contents can have an appearance suggestive of gastroschisis. Location of the umbilical cord insertion and identification of eviscerated organs (see below) can further help to distinguish between these entities.

Evaluation of the Relationship Between the Umbilical Cord and the Defect

When an omphalocele is present, the umbilical cord inserts into the apex of the extra-abdominal

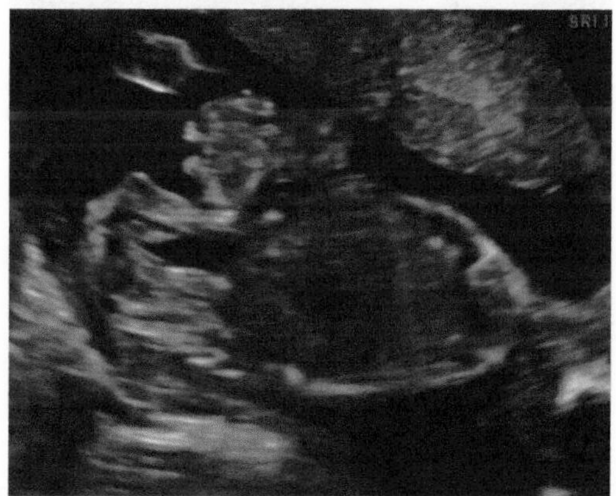

Fig. 2. Sagittal view of a second-trimester fetus with gastroschisis. Note the free-floating loops of bowel in the amniotic cavity.

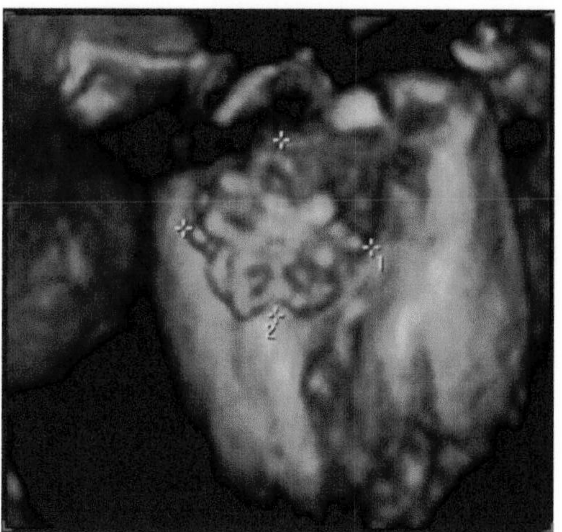

Fig. 3. Three-dimensional image of a second-trimester fetus with gastroschisis. The calipers mark the extra-abdominal loops of bowel, measuring 3.2 × 2.9 cm.

mass (**Fig. 5**). With gastroschisis, the defect is paraumbilical and is almost always located to the right of an otherwise normal-appearing cord insertion (**Fig. 6**).[2] **Fig. 7** depicts a normal cord insertion. An umbilical cord insertion that does not fit these patterns should raise suspicion that another or more complex abnormality may be present. If the umbilical cord inserts into the mass of, rather than adjacent to, an apparent gastroschisis, the possibility of ruptured omphalocele should be considered.[33] In the case of cloacal or bladder extrophy, the defect is most often inferior to the cord insertion (**Fig. 8**). A common finding suggestive of

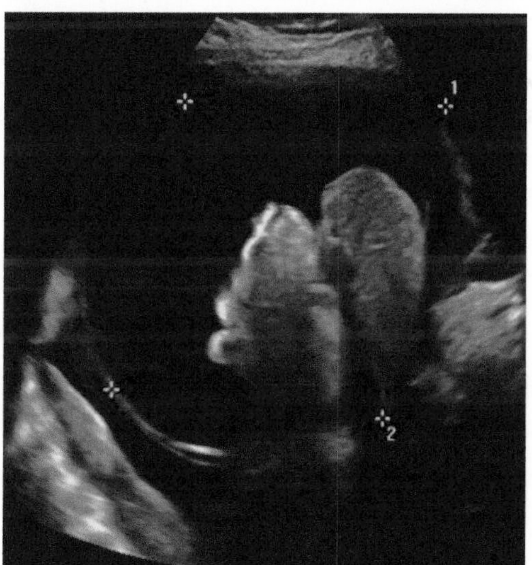

Fig. 4. Omphalocele with ascites. Because of the appearance of freely floating bowel, this could be confused with gastroschisis if the surrounding membrane was not appreciated.

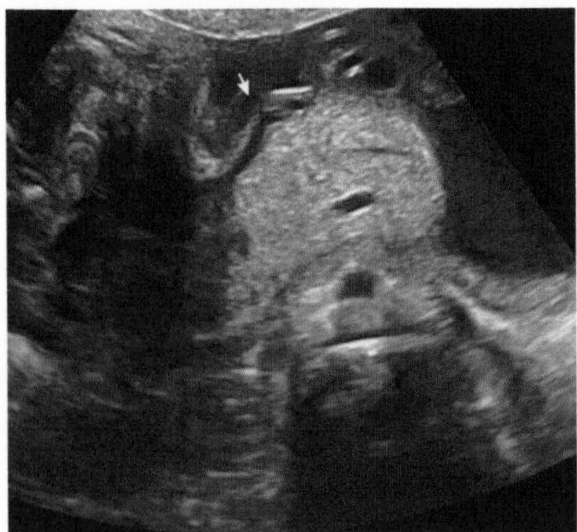

Fig. 5. The arrow marks the cord insertion into the apex of a large omphalocele.

this diagnosis is the absence of a normal-appearing fetal bladder. With cloacal extrophy, there is a complex defect of the inferior abdominal wall that commonly involves an omphalocele as well.[33] When an absent or significantly shortened cord is noted, or the cord seems to be intimately associated with the eviscerated abdominal contents, the possibility of limb–body wall complex should be considered.[5,33–35] This defect involves a number of other anomalies and is discussed further below.

Identification of the Eviscerated Organs

In fetuses with gastroschisis, the majority of cases involve extra-abdominal small bowel; however, the large bowel, stomach, and liver can be involved as well.[3] Herniation of the liver is rare with gastroschisis; however, when present, this finding is

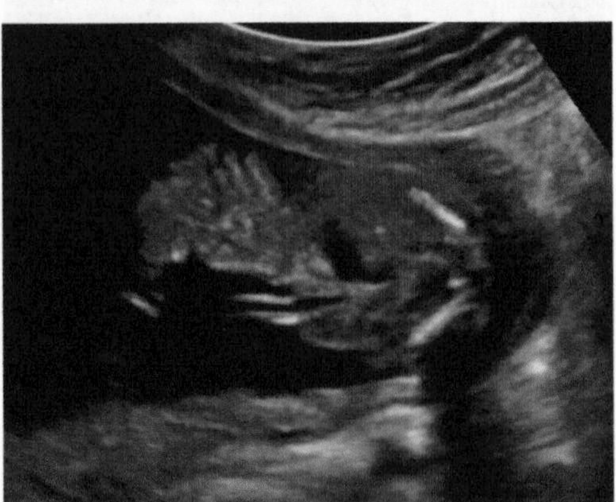

Fig. 6. Transverse abdominal view of a second-trimester fetus with gastroschisis. The right-sided defect is adjacent to the umbilical cord insertion.

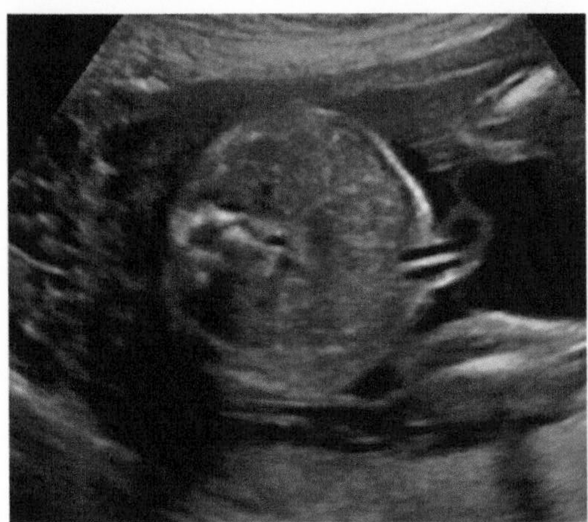

Fig. 7. Normal-appearing umbilical cord insertion in a non-anomalous second-trimester fetus.

associated with high fetal mortality and, among survivors, significant morbidity.[36] Liver herniation in the setting of an apparent gastroschisis should raise suspicion for ruptured omphalocele; as described, characteristics of the cord insertion may help to distinguish these. Similar to gastroschisis, omphaloceles usually contain small bowel alone, although other abdominal organs may be involved (**Figs. 9** and **10**). Location of the liver has several important prognostic implications for pregnancies complicated by omphalocele. As noted, although fetuses with an omphalocele are classically thought to have a high incidence of aneuploidy, this association is strongest when the omphalocele contains small bowel only and

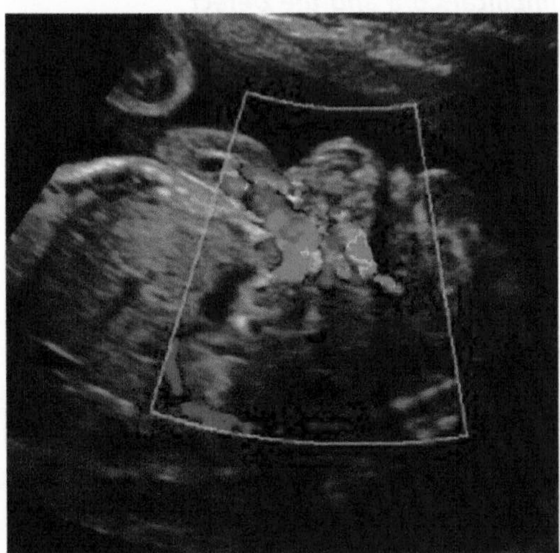

Fig. 8. Sagittal view of a third-trimester fetus with bladder extrophy. The defect is inferior to the umbilical cord insertion (demarcated with color Doppler ultrasonography).

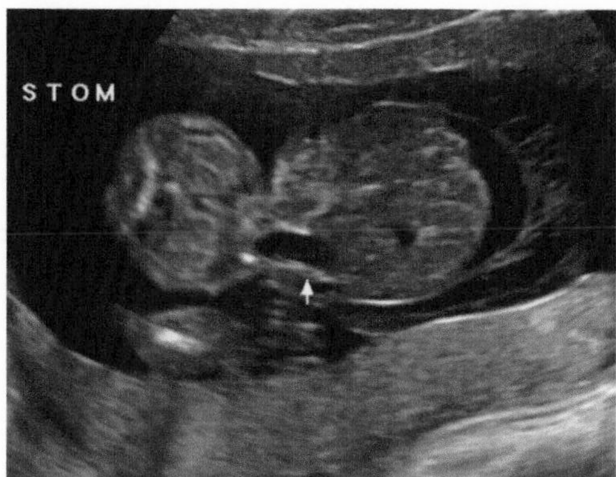

Fig. 9. Transverse abdominal view of a second-trimester fetus with an omphalocele. The arrow marks the herniated fetal stomach.

the liver remains intra-abdominal. A majority of fetuses with liver-containing omphaloceles have a normal karyotype.[34,37–39] Presence or absence of liver within the defect also has implications for postnatal closure. Larger defects, in which the ratio of omphalocele diameter to head circumference was 0.21 or greater, were associated with a higher rate of staged or delayed closure rather than successful primary closure.[40]

Assessment of the Bowel Appearance

With omphalocele, the bowel typically appears normal, despite the abnormal location, because it is protected from the amniotic fluid by the surrounding membrane. It is much more common with gastroschisis to have abnormal-appearing bowel. Bowel can become thickened and/or matted owing to a chemical peritonitis caused by

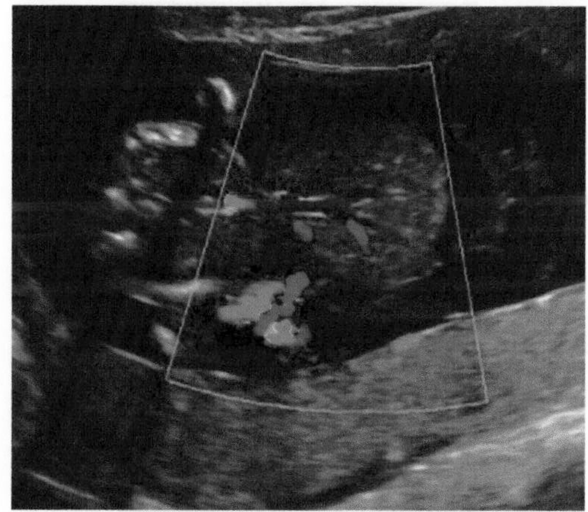

Fig. 10. Transverse abdominal view of a second-trimester fetus with a liver-containing omphalocele. Note the homogeneous appearance of the liver as well as the clearly demarcated extra-abdominal hepatic vasculature.

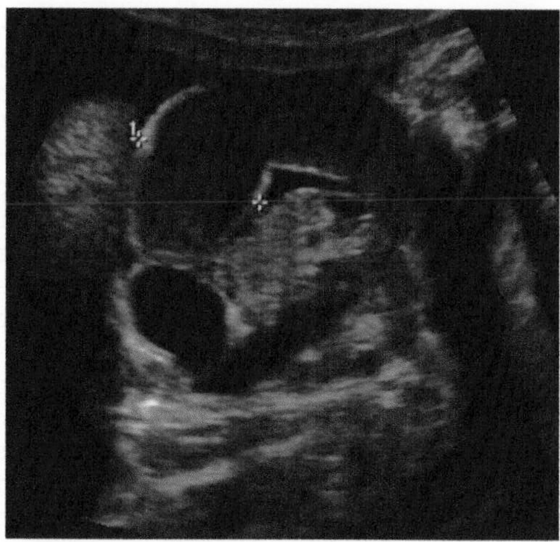

Fig. 11. Dilated loop of extra-abdominal bowel in a third-trimester fetus with gastroschisis. The bowel diameter measures 2.6 cm.

longstanding exposure to amniotic fluid.[2] It is often dilated as well (**Figs. 11** and **12**), which can be a sign of possible obstruction and can lead to perforation. Bowel dilation of greater than 1.8 to 2.0 cm, especially when multiple intra-abdominal dilated loops are present, has been reported to be associated with worse fetal and neonatal outcomes.[33,41–45] The association of gastric dilation with worse neonatal outcome has been reported but not consistently shown.[46,47]

Evaluation for the Presence of Additional Fetal Malformations

This step is extremely important in fetuses with a suspected abdominal wall defect, both for identification of the type of defect as well as determining prognosis. In general, the presence of multiple anomalies, not surprisingly, confers a worse prognosis. Cardiac anomalies are the most common abnormality seen in conjunction with abdominal wall defects. In a review of

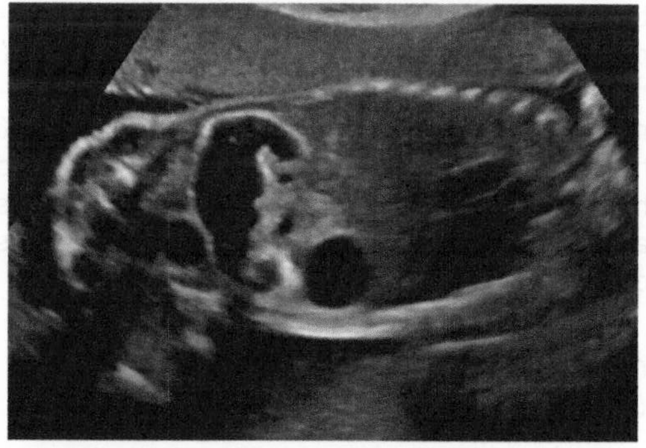

Fig. 12. Dilated loop of intra-abdominal bowel in a third-trimester fetus with gastroschisis.

20 patients with such defects, 47% had congenital heart disease as well.[48] Gastroschisis is typically an isolated anomaly and, in isolation, is not associated with an increased risk of aneuploidy. However, close evaluation for concurrent anomalies should always be performed. In addition to cardiac anomalies, abnormalities of the central nervous system and genitourinary systems, as well as other gastrointestinal malformations, have been found.[2] In contrast with gastroschisis, up to 70% of cases of omphalocele cases are associated with other fetal malformations and up to 40% have a chromosomal abnormality (most commonly trisomies 13, 18, and 21).[2] One series of 37 cases of omphalocele found congenital heart disease in 35% of cases; 69% of these had a normal karyotype.[49]

Extracardiac anomalies may be present as well and could indicate the presence of a syndrome or more complex condition. Beckwith-Wiedemann syndrome should be suspected when an omphalocele is seen in conjunction with fetal macrosomia; hepatic, splenic, and/or renal enlargement; and polyhydramnios.[2,33] Macroglossia is also a common finding with this syndrome; however, this may not be visualized sonographically.[16]

Pentalogy of Cantrell should be suspected when ectopic cordis is seen in conjunction with an omphalocele. The omphalocele associated with pentalogy is often a high defect and may contain the stomach.[2] This diagnosis should be also suspected when a pericardial or pleural effusion is present in a fetus with an omphalocele.[50]

A diagnosis of limb–body wall complex should be considered in cases of a large anterior abdominal wall defect with herniation of the liver, among other abdominal contents, as well as abnormalities of the spine (especially scoliosis), cranium, and extremities (**Figs. 13** and **14**). As mentioned, an absent or shortened umbilical cord is often noted.[2,33–35]

With extrophy of the bladder or a cloaca, a normal-appearing bladder is not seen.[33] Additional anomalies are common with cloacal extrophy; 50% of cases have renal anomalies, 30% have lumbosacral anomalies including meningomyelocele and vertebral anomalies, and 30% have clubbed feet and/or congenitally dislocated hips. The presence of a single umbilical artery is also a common finding. Oligohydramnios is common in the setting of renal abnormalities.[33]

OTHER COMMON PITFALLS AND CHALLENGES

Evaluation of fetal growth is a common challenge when an abdominal wall defect is present. Fetal growth restriction occurs with greater frequency with these conditions, and, not surprisingly, measurement of fetal biometry, specifically the abdominal circumference, is technically challenging when abdominal contents are extra-abdominal. Alternative methods and formulas for estimating fetal weight have been proposed,[51,52] however the standardly-used Hadlock formula seems to be most accurate in making the diagnosis of fetal growth restriction.[53] Our clinical practice is to use the standard formula for estimating fetal weight; we remain cognizant, however, that the abdominal circumference may be underestimated.

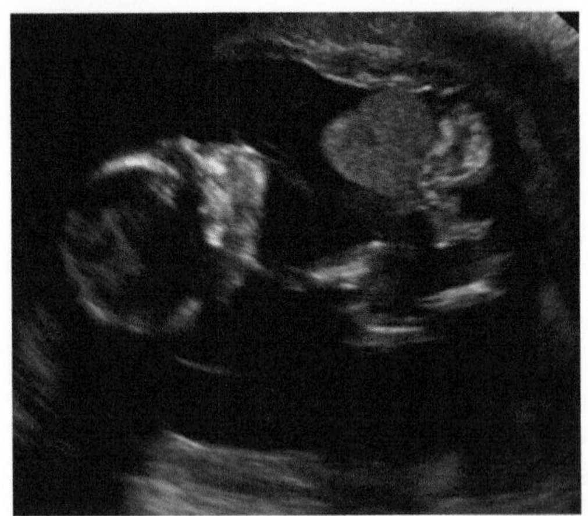

Fig. 13. Sagittal view of first-trimester fetus with limb-body wall complex. Note the herniated abdominal contents in close proximity to the placenta.

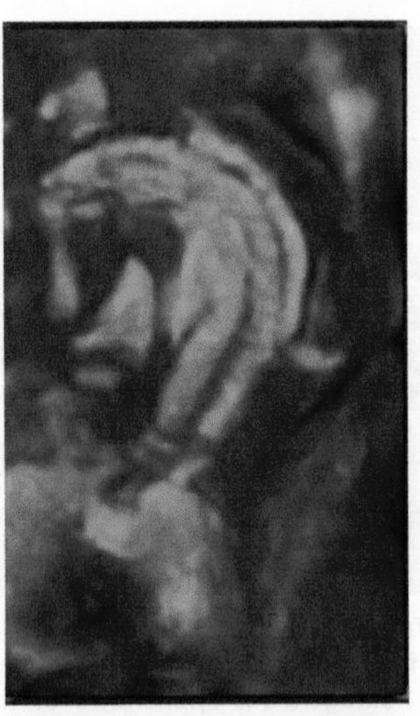

Fig. 14. Three-dimensional image of severe scoliosis in a fetus with limb–body wall complex.

A potential pitfall in making the diagnosis of an abdominal wall defect in the first trimester is confusion with midgut herniation that occurs during normal embryologic development, as discussed. This can be indistinguishable sonographically from a defect in the anterior abdominal wall (see **Fig. 15**). van Zalen-Sprock and colleagues[37] performed serial first-trimester ultrasounds on 18 women with normal pregnancies to characterize the time course of physiologic midgut herniation. They reported that midgut herniation was present in 28% of fetuses at 8 weeks of gestation, 72% at 9 weeks, 100% at 10 weeks, 33% at 11 weeks, and none at 12 weeks. Similar findings have been reported in other studies.[54] Therefore, an abdominal wall defect cannot be diagnosed conclusively until after 12 weeks. An exception to this is if the liver is eviscerated, which does not occur during normal embryologic development.[2,11,34,37]

Other pitfalls include the misdiagnosis of an umbilical hernia or umbilical cord cyst with an omphalocele. In the case of an umbilical cord cyst, there may be a bulging appearance of the anterior abdominal wall; however, all fetal abdominal contents remain intra-abdominal. An umbilical hernia can be distinguished from an omphalocele based on the presence of an intact abdominal wall (subcutaneous fat and skin should not be interrupted).[2] Distinguishing between these entities is important clinically, because umbilical hernias are rarely associated with aneuploidy and they confer a more favorable prognosis in the absence of other anomalies. It is thought that fetal umbilical hernias are a result of an error in normal midgut herniation without the abnormal embryonic disc folding that result in an omphalocele.[55,56]

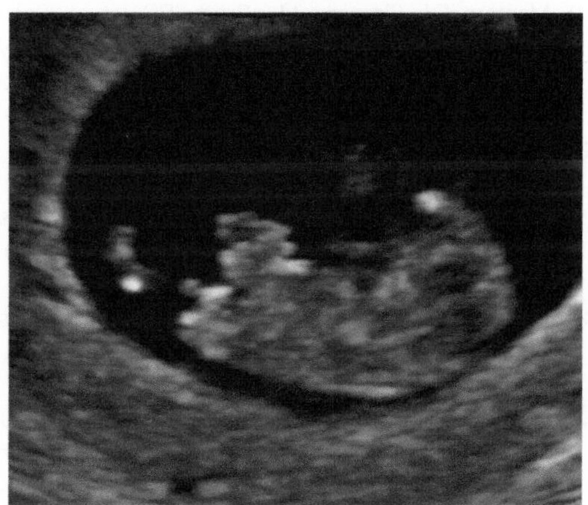

Fig. 15. Physiologic midgut herniation of a fetus at 11 weeks of gestation. This fetus had a normal-appearing abdominal wall at a mid-trimester anatomic survey.

SUMMARY

Congenital abdominal wall defects affect a significant number of pregnancies and are often encountered in obstetric practices. A wide range of abdominal wall defects exist conferring the full spectrum of prognosis and implications for postnatal life. In general, each type of defect has a number of characteristics that allow for reliable sonographic diagnosis, as outlined in this article. Fortunately, the diagnosis is almost always made in the first and second trimesters allowing for options counseling as well as coordination of care with other services to optimize outcomes.

SUPPLEMENTARY DATA

Videos related to this article can be found online at doi:http://dx.doi.org/10.1016/j.cult.2012.08.016.

REFERENCES

1. Syngelaki A, Chelemen T, Dagklis T, et al. Challenges in the diagnosis of fetal non-chromosomal abnormalities at 11-13 weeks. Prenat Diagn 2011; 31:90.
2. Hertzberg BS, Nyberg DA, Neilsen IR. Ventral wall defects. In: Nyberg DA, McGahan JP, Pretorius DH, et al, editors. Diagnostic imaging of fetal anomalies. Philadelphia: Lippincott Williams & Wilkins; 2003. p. 507–46.
3. Duhamel B. Embryology of exomphalos and allied malformations. Arch Dis Child 1963;38:142.
4. Hutchin P. Somatic anomalies of the umbilicus and anterior abdominal wall. Surg Gynecol Obstet 1965;120:1075.
5. Cyr DR, Mack LA, Schoenecker SA, et al. Bowel migration in the normal fetus: US detection. Radiology 1986;161:119.
6. Hoyme HE, Higginbottom MC, Jones KL. The vascular pathogenesis of gastroschisis: intrauterine interruption of the omphalomesenteric artery. J Pediatr Surg 1981;98:228.
7. Hoyme HE, Jones MC, Jones KL. Gastroschisis: abdominal wall disruption secondary to early gestational interruption of the omphalomesenteric artery. Semin Perinatol 1983;7:294.
8. Romero R. Gastroschisis. In: Romero R, Pilu G, Jeanty P, et al, editors. Prenatal diagnosis of congenital anomalies. Norwalk (CT): Appleton & Lange; 1998. p. 224–5.
9. Carpenter MW, Curci MR, Dibbins AW, et al. Perinatal management of ventral wall defects. Obstet Gynecol 1984;64:646.
10. Segel SY, Marder SJ, Parry S, et al. Fetal abdominal wall defects and mode of delivery: a systematic review. Obstet Gynecol 2001;98:867.

11. Bronshtein M, Blazer S, Zimmer EZ. The gastrointestinal tract and abdominal wall. In: Callen PW, editor. Ultrasonography in obstetrics and gynecology. 5th edition. Philadelphia: Saunders Elsevier; 2008. p. 587–639.
12. Margulis L. Omphalocele (amnicele). Am J Obstet Gynecol 1945;49:695.
13. Curtis JA, Watson L. Sonographic diagnosis of omphalocele in the first trimester of fetal gestation. J Ultrasound Med 1988;7:97.
14. Khoury MJ, Erickson JD, Cordero JF, et al. Congenital malformations and intrauterine growth retardation: a population study. Pediatrics 1988;82:83.
15. Nicolaides K, Sebire N, Snijders R. The 11-14 week scan. In: Nicolaides K, editor. The diagnosis of fetal abnormalities. New York: New York; 1999. p. 76–7.
16. Ranzini AC, Day-Salvatore D, Turner T, et al. Intrauterine growth and ultrasound findings in fetuses with Beckwith-Wiedemann syndrome. Obstet Gynecol 1997;89(4):538.
17. Keppler-Noreuil K, Gorton S, Foo F, et al. Prenatal ascertainment of OEIS complex/cloacal exstrophy - 15 new cases and literature review. Am J Med Genet 2007;143A:2122.
18. Bianchi DW, Crombleholme TM, D'Alton ME. Cloacal exstrophy. New York: McGraw-Hill; 2000. p. 459.
19. Sponseller PD, Bisson LJ, Gearhart JP, et al. The anatomy of the pelvis in the exstrophy complex. J Bone Joint Surg Am 1995;77:177.
20. Marshall VF, Muecke EC. Congenital abnormalities of the bladder. In: Handbuch de Urologie. New York: Springer-Verlag; 1968. p. 165.
21. Silver RI, Yang A, Ben-Chaim J, et al. Penile length in adulthood after exstrophy reconstruction. J Urol 1997;157:999.
22. Mathews RI, Gan M, Gearhart JP. Urogynaecological and obstetric issues in women with the exstrophy-epispadias complex. BJU Int 2003;91:845.
23. Bronshtein M, Timor-Tritsch I, Rottem S. Early detection of fetal anomalies. In: Timor-Tritsch I, Rottem S, editors. Transvaginal sonography. New York: Chapman & Hall; 1991. p. 327.
24. Bianchi DW, Crombleholme TM, D'Alton ME. Body-stalk anomaly. In: Fetology. New York: McGraw-Hill; 2000. p. 453.
25. Lockwood CJ, Scioscia AL, Hobbins JC. Congenital absence of the umbilical cord resulting from maldevelopment of embryonic body folding. Am J Obstet Gynecol 1986;155:1049.
26. Ginsberg NE, Cadkin A, Strom C. Prenatal diagnosis of body stalk anomaly in the first trimester of pregnancy. Ultrasound Obstet Gynecol 1997;10:419.
27. Daskalakis G, Sebire NJ, Jurkovic D, et al. Body stalk anomaly at 10-14 weeks of gestation. Ultrasound Obstet Gynecol 1997;10:416.
28. Hiett AK, Devoe LD, Falls DG, et al. Ultrasound diagnosis of a twin gestation with concordant body stalk anomaly. J Reprod Med 1992;37:944.
29. Alphonso N, Venugopal PS, Deshpande R, et al. Complete thoracic ectopia cordis. Eur J Cardiothorac Surg 2003;23:426.
30. Moore K. The cardiovascular system. In: Moore K, editor. The developing human clinically oriented embryology. Philadelphia: WB Saunders Company; 1988. p. 286.
31. Hornberger LK, Colan SD, Lock JE, et al. Outcome of patients with ectopia cordis and significant intracardiac defects. Circulation 1996;94:II32.
32. American Institute of Ultrasound in Medicine. AIUM practice Guideline for the Performance of obstetric ultrasound Examinations. AIUM practice guidelines: obstetric ultrasound. Laurel (MD): The American Institute of Ultrasound in Medicine; 2007.
33. Sanders RC, editor. Structural fetal abnormalities. 2nd edition. St Louis (MO): Mosby; 2002.
34. Monteagudo A. Prenatal sonographic diagnosis of fetal abdominal wall defects. In: Brass VA, editor. Waltham (MA): UpToDate; 2011.
35. Murphy A, Platt LD. First-trimester diagnosis of body stalk anomaly using 2- and 3-dimensional sonography. J Ultrasound Med 2011;30(12):1739–43.
36. McClellan EB, Shew SB, Lee SS, et al. Liver herniation in gastroschisis: incidence and prognosis. J Pediatr Surg 2011;46(11):2115–8.
37. van Zalen-Sprock RM, Vugt JM, van Geijn HP. First-trimester sonography of physiological midgut herniation and early diagnosis of omphalocele. Prenat Diagn 1997;17(6):511.
38. Nyberg DA, Fitzsimmons J, Mack LA, et al. Chromosomal abnormalities in fetuses with omphalocele. Significance of omphalocele contents. J Ultrasound Med 1989;8(6):299.
39. Benacerraf BR, Saltzman DH, Estroff JA, et al. Abnormal karyotype of fetuses with omphalocele: prediction based on omphalocele contents. Obstet Gynecol 1990;75(3):317.
40. Montero FJ, Simpson LL, Brady PC, et al. Fetal omphalocele ratios predict outcomes in prenatally diagnosed omphalocele. Am J Obstet Gynecol 2011;205(3):284.
41. Huh NG, Hirose S, Goldstein RB. Prenatal intraabdominal bowel dilation is associated with postnatal gastrointestinal complications in fetuses with gastroschisis. Am J Obstet Gynecol 2010;202(4):396.
42. Kuleva M, Khen-Dunlop N, Dumez Y, et al. Is complex gastroschisis predictable by prenatal ultrasound? BJOG 2012;119(1):102–9.
43. Contro E, Fratelli N, Okoye B, et al. Prenatal ultrasound in the prediction of bowel obstruction in infants with gastroschisis. Ultrasound Obstet Gynecol 2010;35(6):702–7.
44. Garcia L, Brizot M, Liao A, et al. Bowel dilation as a predictor of adverse outcome in isolated fetal gastroschisis. Prenat Diagn 2010;30(10):964–9.

45. Long AM, Court J, Morabito A, et al. Antenatal diagnosis of bowel dilatation in gastroschisis is predictive of poor postnatal outcome. J Pediatr Surg 2011;46(6):1070–5.
46. Alfaraj MA, Ryan G, Langer JC, et al. Does gastric dilation predict adverse perinatal or surgical outcome in fetuses with gastroschisis? Ultrasound Obstet Gynecol 2011;37(2):202–6.
47. Aina-Mumuney AJ, Fischer AC, Blakemore KJ, et al. A dilated fetal stomach predicts a complicated postnatal course in cases of prenatally diagnosed gastroschisis. Am J Obstet Gynecol 2004;190(5):1326–30.
48. Crawford DC, Chapman MG, Allan LD. Echocardiography in the investigation of anterior abdominal wall defects in the fetus. Br J Obstet Gynaecol 1985;92(10):1034.
49. Fogel M, Copel JA, Cullen MT, et al. Congenital heart disease and fetal thoracoabdominal anomalies: associations in utero and the importance of cytogenetic analysis. Am J Perinatol 1991;8(6):411.
50. Siles C, Boyd PA, Manning N, et al. Omphalocele and pericardial effusion: possible sonographic markers for the pentalogy of Cantrell or its variants. Obstet Gynecol 1996;87(5):840–2.
51. Siemer J, Hilbert A, Hart N, et al. Specific weight formula for fetuses with abdominal wall defects. Ultrasound Obstet Gynecol 2008;31(4):397–400.
52. Honarvar M, Allahyari M, Dehbashi S. Assessment of fetal weight based on ultrasonic femur length after the second trimester. Int J Gynaecol Obstet 2001;73(1):15–20.
53. Nicholas S, Tuuli MG, Dicke J, et al. Estimation of fetal weight in fetuses with abdominal wall defects: comparison of 2 recent sonographic formulas to the Hadlock formula. J Ultrasound Med 2010;29(7):1069–74.
54. Timor-Tritsch IE, Warren WB, Peisner DB, et al. First-trimester midgut herniation: a high-frequency transvaginal sonographic study. Am J Obstet Gynecol 1989;161(3):831–3.
55. Haas J, Achiron R, Barzilay E, et al. Umbilical cord hernias (prenatal diagnosis and natural history). J Ultrasound Med 2011;30(12):1629–32.
56. Achiron R, Soriano D, Lipitz S, et al. Fetal midgut herniation into the umbilical cord: improved definition of ventral abdominal anomaly with the use of transvaginal sonography. Ultrasound Obstet Gynecol 1995;6(4):256–60.
57. Luehr B, Lipsett J, Quinlivan JA. Limb-body wall complex: a case series. J Matern Fetal Neonatal Med 2002;12:132.
58. Shapiro E, Lepor H, Jeffs RD. The inheritance of the exstrophy-epispadias complex. J Urol 1984;132:308.
59. Connolly JA, Peppas DS, Jeffs RD, et al. Prevalence and repair of inguinal hernias in children with bladder exstrophy. J Urol 1995;154:1900.
60. Meizner I, Levy A, Barnhard Y. Cloacal exstrophy sequence: an exceptional ultrasound diagnosis. Obstet Gynecol 1995;86:446.
61. Bianchi DW, Crombleholme TM, D'Alton ME. Omphalocele. In: Fetology. New York: McGraw-Hill; 2000. p. 483.
62. Liang RI, Huang SE, Chang F. Prenatal diagnosis of ectopia cordis at 10 weeks of gestation using two-dimensional and three-dimensional ultrasonography. Ultrasound Obstet Gynecol 1997;10:137.

Ultrasonography for Fetal Hydronephrosis

Tulin Ozcan, MD

KEYWORDS

- Fetal hydronephrosis • Pyelectasis • Bladder obstruction • Reflux
- Ureteropelvic junction obstruction • Lower urinary tract obstruction

KEY POINTS

- Fetal hydronephrosis is seen in approximately 0.1% to 5% of all pregnancies on prenatal ultrasonography.
- Fetal hydronephrosis is most often transient or clinically insignificant.
- Measurement of the maximum renal pelvic anteroposterior diameter in the transverse plane is the most accepted method to define fetal hydronephrosis.
- In general, the likelihood of having a significant renal anomaly correlates with the severity of hydronephrosis.
- Because fetuses with hydronephrosis are at increased risk for Down syndrome and congenital anomalies of the kidney and urinary tract, a comprehensive prenatal evaluation is required for these conditions.
- Fetuses with second-trimester unilateral hydronephrosis should undergo repeat testing in the third trimester at 32 to 34 weeks to assess progression and select those who will benefit most from postnatal testing.

INTRODUCTION

Fetal hydronephrosis (FH) is the dilation of the fetal renal collecting system and is one of the most common abnormalities reported in approximately 0.1% to 5% of all pregnancies on prenatal ultrasonography.[1]

Renal collecting system dilation is a transient physiologic condition in most fetuses; however, it can occasionally be secondary to obstruction or reflux. Identification of predictors useful for differentiating variants of normal from those secondary to obstruction or reflux avoids unnecessary intervention and anxiety and allows reasonable management strategies to be developed in antenatal and postnatal periods to preserve renal function.[2]

Currently, the definition of FH is variable, and the antenatal and postnatal approach for management of FH has not been systematically defined. This review summarizes the available data on the diagnosis and management of FH.

FETAL URINARY TRACT DEVELOPMENT AND APPEARANCE ON ULTRASONOGRAPHY

The human embryo develops 3 sets of kidney systems: the pronephros, mesonephros, and metanephros. The metanephros becomes the definitive kidney. The metanephros forms in the sacral region as a pair of new structures called the metanephric diverticulum or ureteric buds. Ureteric buds penetrate the metanephric mesoderm at around 28 days. Differentiation of the

The author identified no financial or financial affiliations.
Department of Obstetrics and Gynecology, 601 Elmwood Avenue, Box 668, Rochester, NY 14607, USA
E-mail address: Tulin_ozcan@urmc.rochester.edu

Ultrasound Clin 8 (2013) 69–77
http://dx.doi.org/10.1016/j.cult.2012.08.015

ureteric bud to the nephron and metanephric mesenchyme to the collecting system are dependent on the proper induction between those 2 tissues. The fetal kidneys ascend from their pelvic position during weeks 6 to 9 of gestation. The cloaca is divided by the urorectal septum to urogenital sinus anteriorly and the anal canal posteriorly. The upper part of the urogenital sinus between the allantois and the mesonephric ducts differentiates to form the bladder.

Fetal kidneys start urine production at 5 to 8 weeks, with tubular function starting at around 14 weeks. Early in gestation, the amniotic fluid is principally a transudate of the amnion, whereas later it is composed of fetal urine and lung fluid. The amniotic volume becomes principally dependent on urine production at around 16 to 20 weeks.

The kidneys can be visualized by ultrasonography at 11 to 12 weeks, with distinct renal architecture seen by the 20th week. The kidneys initially appear echogenic. The echogenicity decreases with advancing gestation. The corticomedullary differentiation starts at 14 to 15 weeks and should be present after 18 weeks. A renal cortex as echogenic as liver or spleen or less in the second and third trimester with relatively hypoechoic medulla is characteristic of normal corticomedullary differentiation. The fetal bladder can be visualized on ultrasonography at 10 to 14 weeks, and its emptying can be seen at 15 weeks. The ureters are normally not visible.

DEFINITION OF FH ON ULTRASONOGRAPHY

Several systems have been developed to diagnosis and grade the severity of FH. In general, the likelihood of having a significant renal anomaly correlates with the severity of hydronephrosis.[2]

Measurement of the maximum anteroposterior diameter of the renal pelvis in the transverse plane, referred to as renal pelvic diameter (RPD), is the most accepted method for defining FH. Pyelectasis is a term used to define mild RPD between 4 and 10 mm. Several studies have established normative data for fetal renal pelvis size based on gestational age.[3–5] However, there remains a lack of consensus on the threshold RPD that defines clinically significant FH with high likelihood for congenital anomalies of the kidney and urinary tract (CAKUT). Lower cutoffs are more sensitive; however, they are associated with higher false-positive results (**Fig. 1**).[6]

RPD is a measure of collecting system dilatation and does not reflect the extent of hydronephrosis and parenchymal changes such as increased echogenicity, thinning, or caliectasis. The Society of Fetal Urology (SFU) recommends using criteria that are based on the degree of pelvic dilation, presence and number of dilated calyces seen, and the presence and severity of parenchymal atrophy (**Box 1**).[6]

The presence of oligohydramnios after 20 weeks is the most sensitive marker of loss of renal

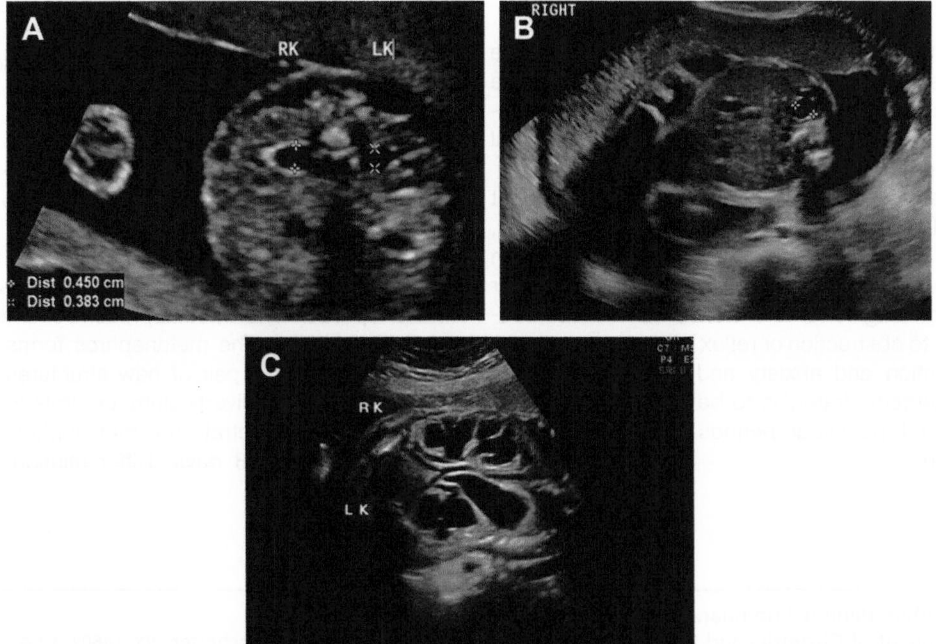

Fig. 1. (*A*) Bilateral mild hydronephrosis with RPD of 4.5 mm and 3.8 mm on the right and left, respectively. (*B*) Unilateral right hydronephrosis of 9.7 mm. (*C*) Severe bilateral hydronephrosis, SFU grade III to IV.

Box 1
SFU criteria for fetal hydronephronisis

- Grade 0: normal examination with no dilatation of the renal pelvis
- Grade 1: mild dilatation of the renal pelvis only
- Grade II: moderate dilatation of the renal pelvis, including a few calyces
- Grade III: dilatation of the renal pelvis with visualization of all the calyces, which are uniformly dilated, and normal renal parenchyma
- Grade IV: similar appearance of the renal pelvis and calyces to grade III plus thinning of the renal parenchyma

function. Other renal findings that indicate loss of function such as loss of or abnormal corticomedullary differentiation, increased echogenicity, the presence of renal cysts, chromosomal anomalies, perinephric urinoma, ureteral dilatation, enlarged renal length, progressive caliectasis, a duplex kidney, or a dilated bladder or other structural anomalies or chromosomal aberrations increase the risk of CAKUT and mortality related to CAKUT.[7] An enlarged fetal bladder and the severity of bladder enlargement are associated with poor outcomes, such as posterior urethral valves (PUVs), megaureters, or prune-belly syndrome with megacystitis.[8]

Most investigators use values more than 4 to 5 mm and 7 to 8 mm as the lowest cutoff for FH in the second and third trimester, respectively. The risk of persistent postnatal hydronephrosis is positively correlated with severity of FH and inversely correlated with gestational age. For example, at 20 weeks' gestation, 18% of fetuses with mean RPD of 6 mm were estimated to have persistent postnatal renal pelvic dilation, compared with 95% of fetuses with 12 mm RPD.[9] Other than gestational age, maternal hydration and the degree of bladder distention may affect the RPD.[10,11]

In general, RPD greater than 10 mm is associated with an increased risk of significant CAKUT. This finding was shown in a meta-analysis classifying FH according to second-trimester and third-trimester RPD measurements to mild, moderate, and severe categories (**Box 2**). The risk of any postnatal disease per degree of FH was 11.9% for mild, 45.1% for moderate, and 88.3% for severe cases.[12]

Exceptions to this rule include vesicoureteral reflux (VUR) and decreasing hydronephrosis with loss of renal function and urine production in lower urinary tract obstruction (LUTO) such as PUVs.

Box 2
Categories of hydronephrosis

- Mild hydronephrosis defined as ≤7 mm in the second trimester or ≤9 mm in the third trimester
- Moderate hydronephrosis defined as 7–10 mm in the second trimester or 9–15 mm in the third trimester
- Severe hydronephrosis defined as >10 mm in the second trimester or >15 mm in the third trimester

VUR can be seen in any severity of FH, including resolution in pregnancy. However, VUR associated with mild to moderate FH of RPD less than 15 mm does not seem to cause significant scarring or be a reliable predictor of renal damage in pediatric patients hospitalized with urinary tract infections (UTIs).[9]

ETIOLOGY OF FETAL HYDRONEPHROSIS

FH may develop secondary to transient dilation of the collecting system, upper urinary tract obstruction, nonobstructive processes such as VUR, megaureters, multicystic dysplastic kidney (MCDK), and LUTO caused by ureteroceles, ectopic ureter, PUVs, and urethral atresia, megacystis-microcolon-intestinal hypoperistalsis (MMIH) and prune-belly syndrome. The most common causes are transient hydronephrosis in 41% to 88%, ureteropelvic junction (UPJ) obstruction in 10% to 30%, and VUR in 10% to 20%.[6]

Transient hydronephrosis is related either to physiologic inability to concentrate urine in fetuses or to a transient narrowing of the UPJ early in development, which resolves as the fetus matures.[6] Mild hydronephrosis with RPD less than 6 mm in the second trimester or less than 8 mm in the third trimester is usually associated with transient hydronephrosis, whereas in moderate to severe cases, the incidence of transient hydronephrosis is lower.[13]

Fetal UPJ obstruction refers to distention of the fetal renal pelvis and calyces with urine caused by functional or anatomic obstruction of the ureter. The male/female ratio is 2 to 4:1, with two-thirds of obstructions occurring on the left side. The obstruction is bilateral in 10% to 40% of fetuses. Type I UPJ obstruction is a primary defect at the UPJ, which can be caused by a ureteral stricture, aberrant insertion of the ureter into the renal pelvis, a congenital ureteral fold, a hypoplastic ureteral segment, or an adynamic (but macroscopically normal) UPJ. Most cases of UPJ obstruction are caused by these intrinsic abnormalities. Type II UPJ obstruction is a result of defects occurring secondary to VUR, which leads to progressive elongation of the ureter and kinking at its attachment to the fetal kidney.[14]

There is an increased incidence of other urologic abnormalities, such as VUR and MCDK, with UPJ obstruction.[6] Randomized trials suggest that 19% to 25% of children with prenatally diagnosed UPJ obstruction require surgical intervention.

VUR is the retrograde flow of urine from the bladder into the ureters and renal pelvis. The cause of primary VUR is a developmental anomaly resulting in an inadequate length of the intravesical submucosal ureter. Secondary VUR is associated with LUTO such as PUVs. An international grading system consists of 5 grades for VUR, with increasing severity from grade 1 to grade 5. VUR has a natural tendency to resolve as the intravesical part of the ureter lengthens with growth, and by age 10 years about 75% of VUR cases resolve. Rate of resolution is faster in males and slowest in those with the highest grades. Dilating reflux (grades 3–5) has been shown to be significantly associated with reflux nephropathy secondary to recurrent UTIs and parenchymal scarring caused by severe reflux.[15] Associated urologic anomalies are seen in 13% to 30%. Coexistence of reflux with other renal anomalies increases the risk of reflux nephropathy to 50%.[16,17]

Megaureter refers to a dilated ureter with or without dilation of the renal pelvis and calyces. The presence of calicectasis or pelviectasis is dependent on the duration and severity of the obstruction. Megaureter is classified as obstructive type (ureterovesical junction obstruction), refluxing type (VUR from functional problems at the ureterovesical junction or bladder outlet obstruction) and nonobstructive, nonrefluxing type. The obstructive or refluxing types are categorized as primary or secondary. In primary obstructive megaureter, the obstruction is most commonly caused by functional obstruction at the level of the ureterovesical junction. Primary obstructive megaureter occurs 3.5 to 5 times more often in males. It is 2-fold to 3-fold more common on the left side and is bilateral in 15% to 25 % of patients. In children with FH, the incidence of primary megaureters is approximately 5% to 10%. Most (up to 72%) spontaneously resolve during postnatal follow-up.[6]

MCDK is a severe form of cystic renal dysplasia in which the kidney consists of a group of cysts representing immature nephrons, without any identifiable renal tissue. The primary defect leading to this malformation is an abnormality of the ureteral bud, leading to atresia or absence of the ureter. MCDK is the most common renal cystic disease, is a frequent cause of infantile abdominal masses, and is the second most common prenatally detected urinary tract abnormality.[18] Failure of urine production eventually causes the cysts to shrink. MCDK can develop secondary to early severe urinary tract obstruction and can be segmental.

The severity of renal dysplasia is proportional to the degree of ureteric obstruction. The classic type has a random configuration of noncommunicating cysts, which may be difficult to differentiate from FH. A hydronephrotic type of MCDK has been defined that presents with a discernible, dilated renal pelvis surrounded by cysts.[19] Hydronephrotic and segmental MCDK may be difficult to differentiate from FH alone.

A ureterocele is a cystic dilation of the distal part of the ureter located either within the bladder or spanning the bladder neck and urethra. An ectopic ureter is an abnormally located terminal portion of the ureter. Instead of entering the trigonal area of the bladder, the ureter opens in the urethra, vagina, or uterus. In females, the ectopic ureter may enter from the bladder neck to the perineum and into the vagina, uterus, and even rectum. In males, the ectopic ureter always enters the urogenital system above the external sphincter or pelvic floor and usually into the vas deferens, seminal vesicles, or ejaculatory duct. Ureterocele and ectopic ureter are commonly associated with a double collecting system. In double collecting systems, ureteroceles typically originate from the upper pole of the kidney, and the upper pole ureter is the ectopic ureter as a rule. Ureterocele, ectopic ureters, and duplex systems are often readily identified on prenatal ultrasonography, accounting for 5% to 7% of cases with FH.[6]

PUVs are tissue leaflets fanning distally from the prostatic urethra to the external urinary sphincter. PUV almost exclusively affects male fetuses, with an incidence of 1 in 5000 to 8000 male births. More than half of LUTO cases are caused by PUV. The timing of in utero obstruction predicts the severity of renal dysplasia and overall outcome. Neonatal death is often secondary to pulmonary dysplasia as a result of chronic, early-onset oligohydramnios. Perinatal mortality is as high as 90% to 95% if second-trimester oligohydramnios is present. With obstruction in the third trimester, renal changes may be limited to hydronephrosis alone.

Total obstruction causes distention of the bladder (megacystis) and leads to VUR and hydronephrosis. Reflux, in turn, may cause megaureter (secondary refluxing type).

LUTO carries a worse prognosis, with increased mortality and morbidity because of pulmonary hypoplasia and renal damage compared with the commonly unilateral upper urinary tract obstruction.[20] LUTO diagnosed during the first and second trimester is equally likely from PUV or varying degrees of urethral atresia.[21] However, the earlier the prenatal diagnosis of LUTO is made, the more likely it is to be associated with urethral atresia.[22]

Urethral atresia is the most severe form of obstructive uropathy in boys and refers to maldevelopment of the urethra. Urethral atresia is nearly always fatal unless the urachus remains patent throughout gestation. If the urachus is patent, oligohydramnios is unlikely and the infant usually survives. Prune-belly syndrome can accompany the presentation in some cases. Urethral reconstruction is difficult, and most patients are managed with urinary diversion.

MMIH is most commonly observed in females. MMIH syndrome is a combination of a distended unobstructed bladder, dilated small bowel, and distal microcolon. Gastric and intestinal motility are impaired and this is believed to be related to an intrinsic abnormality of the smooth muscle gene. The small bowel is short, dilated, and malfixed, without an anatomic obstruction in most patients. Microcolon is a transient finding, possibly because of hypoperistalsis. The colon size is normal or dilated in fetuses who survive.

Prune-belly syndrome is a rare congenital anomaly characterized by partial or complete absence of abdominal wall musculature, urinary tract malformation, and in males, cryptorchidism. It is caused by urethral obstruction early in development, leading to massive bladder distention and urinary ascites, and degeneration of the abdominal wall musculature and failure of testicular descent. Prune-belly syndrome exists almost exclusively in males and has an estimated incidence of 1 in 35,000 to 1 in 50,000 live births.[23]

FETAL HYDRONEPROSIS AND DOWN SYNDROME

Mild hydronephrosis is a common finding in fetuses with Down syndrome. RPD of 4 mm or greater is noted in 18% of fetuses with Down syndrome compared with 0% to 3% in normal fetuses. A detailed anatomic examination and search for Down syndrome ultrasonographic markers are indicated in FH. The incidence of Down syndrome is low in women with no other risk factors such as advanced maternal age and other ultrasonographic anomalies and negative serum screen; thus, genetic amniocentesis is not justified in this population.[24]

ULTRASONOGRAPHIC EXAMINATION

Once FH is detected, a detailed anatomic examination and assessment of the genitourinary system should be performed. The severity of FH should be quantitated using both RPD and the SFU criteria. Bilateral FH increases the risk of a significant renal abnormality and the risk of impaired postnatal renal function. Thinning of the renal parenchyma, abnormal or absent corticomedullary differentiation, and presence of cortical cysts indicate injury or impaired development of the renal cortex. Oligohydramnios is consistent with impaired renal function, resulting in a decreased production of fetal urine (amniotic fluid).

When ureters are not visible, the condition is most likely consistent with either transient FH or UPJ obstruction (**Fig. 2**). UPJ obstruction is characterized by varying degrees of fetal renal pelvic dilatation, caliectasis, no visible ipsilateral ureter, a normal bladder, and normal amniotic fluid volume and absence of ectopic ureterocele, or urethral dilation. The characteristic sonographic features of caliceal dilation are multiple parenchymal cystic structures of uniform size with communication between the cysts. Dysplastic changes in the kidneys are rare. A fluid-filled sac posterior to a decompressed, and often dysplastic kidney is seen in severe cases after rupture with urinoma formation.

The differential diagnosis of ureteric dilatation with FH includes VUR, megaureter, PUV, prune-belly syndrome, and ectopic ureter. In VUR, dilation of the renal pelvis and ureters is usually bilateral. The dilation may fluctuate during the

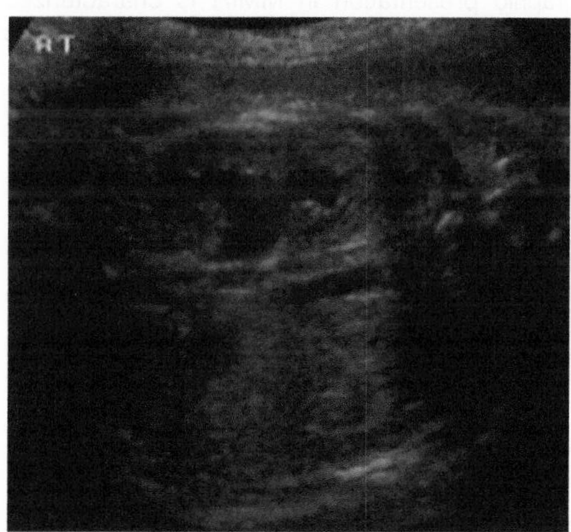

Fig. 2. Right UPJ obstruction.

examination. The dilated pelvis can be traced down to the ureter, with ballooning of the renal pelvis and peristalsis of the dilated ureter when the bladder empties. The bladder may also be enlarged as a result of incomplete emptying. Variably severe hydronephrosis during serial ultrasonographic examinations is typical and is attributed to voiding, which induces reflux.[25]

The combination of prenatal hydronephrosis, ureteral dilation and a normal bladder suggests a megaureter (**Fig.** 3A). Megaureters can be refluxing, obstructed (ureterovesical junction obstruction), nonrefluxing/nonobstructed, and refluxing/obstructed. Most common types are secondary to reflux only and nonrefluxing nonobstructed.

Increased thickness and trabeculation of the bladder wall are consistent with urinary tract obstruction distal to the bladder (LUTO). The most common cause of bladder obstruction in the neonate is PUVs, but other obstructive disorders include urethral atresia, obstructing ureterocele, persistent cloaca, megalourethra, megacystis microcolon syndrome (MMIH), or prune-belly syndrome (**Fig.** 4A–C). Antenatal differentiation between these disorders and PUV may not always be possible. The keyhole sign, representing a dilatation of the posterior urethra in patients with posterior urethral obstruction, is believed to be a specific sign of PUV. However, the keyhole sign is present in 35% of fetuses with bilateral hydronephrosis from other causes, including 50% of the fetuses who had reflux diagnosed postnatally, and is present in only 50% of fetuses with PUV.[26]

Sex determination is a crucial diagnostic step, because PUV primarily occurs in male fetuses and is rare in females. The causes of LUTOs in females are agenesis of the urethra, MMIH syndrome, and persistent cloaca. The ultrasonographic presentation in MMIH is characterized by dilated loops of bowel and polyhydramnios caused by bowel obstruction. Fetuses with prune-belly syndrome have ureteric dilation that is proportionally greater than expected for the RPD, an enlarged bladder with evidence of a urachal abnormality, and megaurethra, with usually normal amniotic fluid volume.

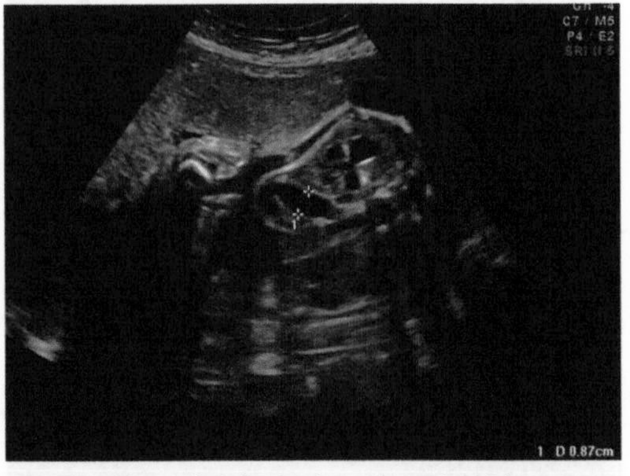

Fig. 3. Unilateral right hydronephrosis with ureteromegaly measuring 8.7 mm.

One study investigating prenatal sonographic differential diagnosis of bladder distention and pyelectasis reported that oligohydramnios, progressive bladder wall thickening, and a dilated posterior urethra were most suggestive of PUVs, whereas a patent urachus was more consistent with prune-belly syndrome. Pyelectasis and megacystis without associated amniotic fluid, bladder, urethral, or renal abnormalities correlated with VUR. However, there was overlap in the findings: oligohydramnios was present in 8 of 10 cases of PUV as well as in 1 of 4 cases of prune-belly syndrome; a dilated posterior urethra was observed in 7 of 10 cases of PUV and transiently in 2 of 4 cases of prune-belly syndrome; bladder wall thickening was present in all cases of PUV and in 2 of 4 patients with prune-belly syndrome.[27]

The classic presentation of MCDK is a multiloculated abdominal mass consisting of multiple noncommunicating thin-walled cysts. On the contrary, the cysts in FH communicate with the enlarged renal pelvis. The reniform shape is preserved with FH, whereas in MCDK the cysts are distributed randomly and the kidney is usually enlarged, with an irregular outline. No renal pelvis or ureter can be shown. Circumferential cysts and a dilated pelvic may be seen with segmental MCDK or MCDK secondary to LUTO.

The sonographic findings of simple ureterocele include hydronephrosis, whereas a duplex system ureterocele shows a dilated upper pole, with 2 noncommunicating collecting systems. The bladder is enlarged if the ureterocele interferes with voiding and the ipsilateral kidney may be obstructed (**Fig. 5**). Ureterocele may be missed with a full or empty fetal bladder.

Urinoma is a fluid mass formed by extravasated urine encapsulated in the perirenal fascia. Urinomas are secondary to urinary obstruction such as PUVs or UPJ obstruction. Urinary ascites can be secondary to spontaneous or iatrogenic rupture of the bladder and the renal calices because of lower obstruction and increased pressure, or rarely because of neurogenic bladder (**Fig. 6**).

MANAGEMENT

Management is based on the presence of extrarenal and other renal anomalies, amount of amniotic fluid volume, gestational age, severity

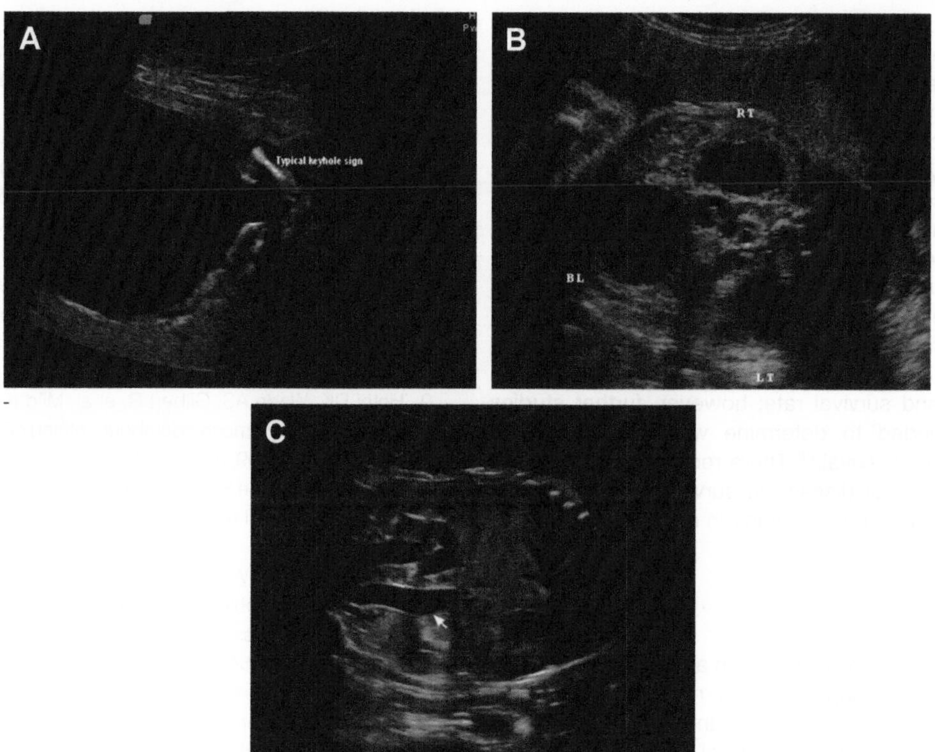

Fig. 4. (*A*) Keyhole sign. (*B*) PUV and bilateral hydronephrosis with thickened bladder walls. (*C*) Same patient as (*B*), with bilateral ureteromegaly (*arrow*).

of hydronephrosis, and whether the FH is unilateral versus bilateral.

Because mild hydronephrosis serves as a weak marker for Down syndrome, assessment of the fetal karyotype should be offered if additional fetal anomalies are detected, in women of advanced maternal age, and in women with abnormal maternal serum screening tests for Down syndrome.

Fetuses with unilateral mild hydronephrosis should have a follow-up ultrasonographic scan at 32 to 34 weeks. Those with resolution have a low risk of clinically significant disease, whereas RPD greater than 7 to 8 mm at this gestational age is an indication for postnatal evaluation.

Moderately severe FH, solitary kidney or bilaterality, progression on serial examinations, presence of oligohydramnios, renal dysplastic changes such

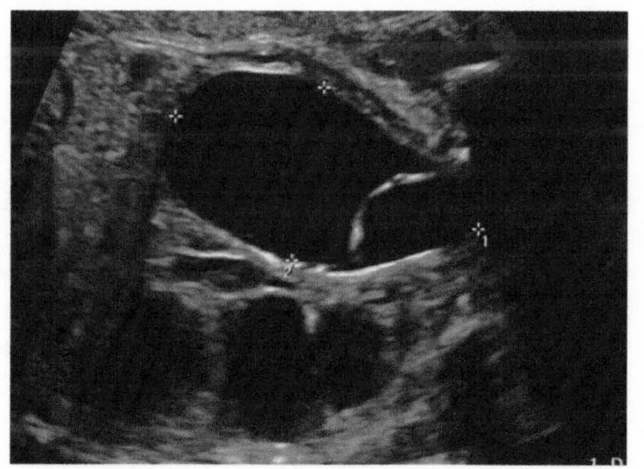

Fig. 5. Obstructing ureterocele with enlarged bladder.

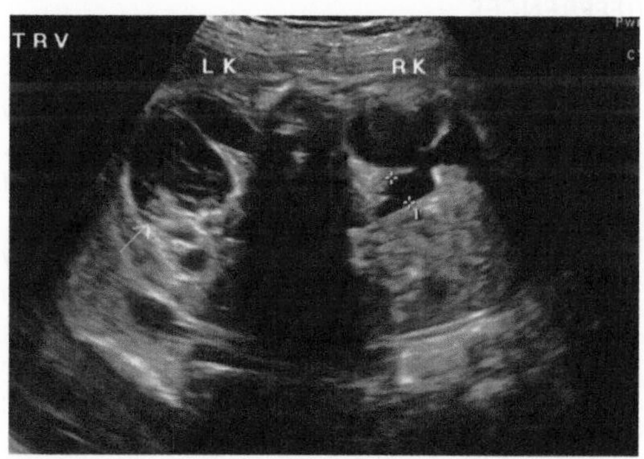

Fig. 6. Bilateral hydronephrosis, urinoma on the left kidney secondary to PUV (*white arrow*) and dilated ureter (*calipers*) with hydronephrosis on the right side.

as hyperechogenicity or renal cysts, thickened bladder wall, ureteromegaly, presence of urinoma, or urinary ascite necessitate close follow-up every 2 to 3 weeks to assess progression and amniotic fluid volumes.

Early delivery has been suggested for fetuses with severe oligohydramnios and documented lung maturity and may be indicated to reduce the risk of other adverse outcomes from oligohydramnios such as umbilical cord compression.

Antenatal bladder drainage by a vesicoamniotic shunt for LUTO may increase the amount of amniotic fluid, thus potentially improving lung development and survival rate; however, further studies are needed to determine whether intervention improves survival.[28] There remains a high rate of chronic renal disease in survivors, necessitating renal replacement therapy in almost two-thirds of cases.

SUMMARY

FH is a common problem on antenatal ultrasonography. The diagnosis and management of FH are based on an understanding of the cause, pathophysiology, and natural history. Most cases are transient and clinically insignificant. In fetuses with increased RPD, ultrasonographic study should assess for the presence of other anomalies, oligohydramnios, bilateralism, caliectasis, parenchymal echogenicity, parenchymal thinning, presence of bladder and ureter enlargement, and bladder wall thickness, which, if present, increase the risk of CAKUT. In utero management for LUTO by placement of vesicoamniotic shunts increases survival, but there is significant risk of long-term severe renal impairment. The impact of early delivery for oligohydramnios has not been extensively studied and remains unknown.

REFERENCES

1. Sidhu G, Beyene J, Rosenblum ND. Outcome of isolated antenatal hydronephrosis: a systematic review and meta-analysis. Pediatr Nephrol 2006;21:218–24.
2. Woodward M, Frank D. Postnatal management of antenatal hydronephrosis. BJU Int 2002;89:149–56.
3. Chitty LS, Altman DG. Charts of fetal size: kidney and renal pelvis measurements. Prenat Diagn 2003;23:891–7.
4. Scott JE, Wright B, Wilson G, et al. Measuring the fetal kidney with ultrasonography. Br J Urol 1995; 76:769–74.
5. Odibo AO, Raab E, Elovitz M, et al. Prenatal mild pyelectasis: evaluating the thresholds of renal pelvic diameter associated with normal postnatal renal function. J Ultrasound Med 2004;23:513–7.
6. Nguyen HT, Herndon CD, Cooper C, et al. The society for fetal urology consensus statement on the evaluation and management of antenatal hydronephrosis. J Pediatr Urol 2010;6:212–31.
7. Maizels M, Wang E, Sabbagha RE, et al. Late second trimester assessment of pyelectasis (SERP) to predict pediatric urological outcome is improved by checking additional features. J Matern Fetal Neonatal Med 2006;19:295–303.
8. Maizels M, Alpert SA, Houston JT, et al. Fetal bladder sagittal length: a simple monitor to assess normal and enlarged fetal bladder size, and forecast clinical outcome. J Urol 2004;172:1995–9.
9. Hothi DK, Wade AS, Gilbert R, et al. Mild fetal renal pelvis dilatation: much ado about nothing? Clin J Am Soc Nephrol 2009;4(1):168–77.
10. Robinson JN, Tice K, Kolm P, et al. Effect of maternal hydration on fetal renal pyelectasis. Obstet Gynecol 1998;92:137–41.
11. Leung VY, Chu WC, Metreweli C. Hydronephrosis index: a better physiological reference in antenatal ultrasound for assessment of fetal hydronephrosis. J Pediatr 2009;154:116–20.
12. Lee RS, Cendron M, Kinnamon DD, et al. Antenatal hydronephrosis as a predictor of postnatal outcome: a meta-analysis. Pediatrics 2006;118: 586–93.
13. Mallik M, Watson AR. Antenatally detected urinary tract abnormalities: more detection but less action. Pediatr Nephrol 2008;23:897–904.
14. Hanna MK. Antenatal hydronephrosis and ureteropelvic junction obstruction: the case for early intervention. Urology 2000;55:612–5.
15. Blumenthal I. Vesicoureteric reflux and urinary tract infection in children. Postgrad Med J 2006;82: 31–5.
16. Hunziker M, Kutasy B, D'Asta F, et al. Urinary tract anomalies associated with high grade primary vesicoureteral reflux. Pediatr Surg Int 2012;28: 201–4.
17. Anderson PA, Rickwood AM. Features of primary vesicoureteral reflux detected by prenatal sonography. Br J Urol 1991;67:267–71.
18. Al-Ghwery S, Al-Asmar A. Multicystic dysplastic kidney: conservative management and follow-up. Ren Fail 2005;27:189–92.
19. Rizzo N, Gabrielli S, Pilu G, et al. Prenatal diagnosis and obstetrical management of multicystic dysplastic kidney disease. Prenat Diagn 1987;7: 109–18.
20. Peters CA, Reid LM, Docimo S, et al. The role of the kidney in lung growth and maturation in the setting of obstructive uropathy and oligohydramnios. J Urol 1991;146(21):597–600.
21. Robyr R, Benachi A, Daikha-Dahmane F, et al. Correlation between ultrasound and anatomical findings in fetuses with lower urinary tract obstruction in

the first half of pregnancy. Ultrasound Obstet Gynecol 2005;25:478–82.
22. Sebire N, Kaisenberg CV, Rubio C, et al. Fetal megacystis at 10–14 weeks of gestation. Ultrasound Obstet Gynecol 1996;8:387–90.
23. Tonni G, Ida V, Alessandro V, et al. Prune-belly syndrome: case series and review of the literature regarding early prenatal diagnosis, epidemiology, genetic factors, treatment, and prognosis. Fetal Pediatr Pathol 2012. [Epub ahead of print].
24. Coco C, Jeanty P. Isolated fetal pyelectasis and chromosomal abnormalities. Am J Obstet Gynecol 2005;193:732–8.
25. Anderson NG, Allan RB, Abbott GD. Fluctuating fetal or neonatal renal pelvis: marker of high-grade vesicoureteral reflux. Pediatr Nephrol 2004;19: 749–53.
26. Bernardes LS, Aksnes G, Saada J, et al. Keyhole sign: how specific is it for the diagnosis of posterior urethral valves? Ultrasound Obstet Gynecol 2009; 34:419–23.
27. Montemarano H, Bulas DI, Rushton HG, et al. Bladder distention and pyelectasis in the male fetus: causes, comparisons, and contrasts. J Ultrasound Med 1998;17:743–6.
28. Morris RK, Malin GL, Khan KS, et al. Systematic review of the effectiveness of antenatal intervention for the treatment of congenital lower urinary tract obstruction. BJOG 2010;117: 382–90.

Ultrasound for Evaluation of Fetal Anemia

Eva K. Pressman, MD

KEYWORDS

• Fetal anemia • Alloimmunization • Fetal transfusion • Middle cerebral artery Dopplers
• Hydrops fetalis

KEY POINTS

- Fetal anemia is a treatable cause of hydrops fetalis.
- Middle cerebral artery Doppler velocimetry can predict significant fetal anemia.
- Intrauterine transfusion can successfully treat fetal anemia caused by alloimmunization, fetomaternal hemorrhage, and parvovirus infection, and some cases of twin–twin transfusion or fetal hemoglobinopathies.

 **Video of transfusion into the placental insertion of the umbilical vein with an anterior placenta accompanies this article.**

BACKGROUND

Fetal anemia and resultant hydrops fetalis was first described more than 400 years ago and a description was first published by Ballantine[1,2] in late 1800s. Since then, great advances have been made in the diagnosis and treatment of fetal anemia. Management of fetal anemia relies on appropriate suspicion based on clinical history or sonographic findings, application of both invasive and noninvasive diagnostic technologies, and a combination of in utero therapy, delivery planning, and postnatal management. As with most conditions, an understanding of the cause and natural history of the fetal anemia can guide the most effective management strategy.

CAUSES OF FETAL ANEMIA

Fetal anemia can result from increased destruction, abnormal production, or other loss of fetal red blood cells. Increased destruction is most often caused by alloimmunization, whereas abnormal production can be related to hemoglobinopathies or viral bone marrow suppression. Loss of red cells from the fetal circulation can also occur through fetomaternal hemorrhage, twin–twin transfusion, or bleeding within the fetus from trauma, vascular malformation, or a coagulation abnormality. In all of these cases, the end result is fetal anemia, and management often involves transfusion, either before or after delivery.

Alloimmunization

The most common cause of fetal anemia is alloimmunization. Rhesus (Rh) D antibodies were first associated with fetal death in 1939 by Levine and Stetson[3] in a patient who had a stillbirth and then experienced a severe hemolytic reaction to transfusion of her husband's blood. Over the next decade, advances were made in neonatal treatment with exchange transfusions. In the early 1960s, assessment of fetal risk through evaluating amniotic fluid for evidence of hemolysis was

Disclosures: None.
Funding: None.
Department of Obstetrics and Gynecology, University of Rochester, 601 Elmwood Avenue, Box 668, Rochester, NY 14642, USA
E-mail address: eva_pressman@urmc.rochester.edu

Ultrasound Clin 8 (2013) 79–87
http://dx.doi.org/10.1016/j.cult.2012.08.009
1556-858X/13/$ – see front matter

described.[4] In 1963, the first successful fetal intraperitoneal transfusion for Rh sensitization was described.[5] This approach was tried after a similar intraperitoneal transfusion technique had been used for the treatment of sickle cell anemia in neonates in Africa and led to replenishment of intravascular red cells. The procedure was performed with radiographic guidance after instillation of intraamniotic contrast that was swallowed by the fetus and used to outline the fetal intestines.

The process of amniotic fluid assessment for hemolysis followed by intraperitoneal transfusion under radiographic or fluoroscopic guidance continued through the next 2 decades, although the introduction of Rh immune globulin in the late 1960s decreased the incidence of Rh D sensitization markedly. The approach to intrauterine assessment and fetal treatment changed significantly in the 1980s with the introduction of ultrasound. Real-time ultrasound not only allowed better assessment of the fetus but also markedly improved the ability to treat the fetus in utero.

Despite the ability to prevent Rh D sensitization with Rh D immunoglobulin, the condition still occurs because of missed or inadequate immune prophylaxis. In addition, alloimmunization to other blood surface antigens now accounts for a large percentage of cases. These blood surface antigens include others in the Rh family (c, C, e, and E), Kell, and numerous other minor antigens. Although all of these antigens can lead to immune destruction of fetal red cells, Kell antigens also have been associated with erythropoietic suppression.[6] This condition leads to significantly greater degree of fetal anemia for a given antibody titer and also leads to underestimation of fetal anemia based on assessment of amniotic fluid assessment for bilirubin. Middle cerebral artery (MCA) Doppler peak systolic velocity seems to offer the best assessment for anemia in the Kell-sensitized fetus[7]

Viral Infection

Many congenital viral infections have been associated with hydrops fetalis, but only parvovirus B19 has been specifically associated with fetal anemia and, even more importantly, anemia amenable to treatment by intrauterine transfusion. Although 30% to 50% of pregnant women are susceptible to parvovirus infection, only 1% to 2% will seroconvert during pregnancy and less than a third of these will transmit the virus to the fetus.[8] The risk of hydrops with fetal parvovirus infection is caused not only by inhibition of erythropoiesis but also possibly by hypoalbuminemia, hepatitis, myocarditis, and placentitis.[8] Although the disease is self-limited and even hydropic fetuses have been seen to improve without treatment, if severe anemia is suspected or progresses, intrauterine transfusion has been shown to lead to good outcomes.

Hemorrhage

Fetal hemorrhage includes bleeding into the fetus itself, through the placenta into the maternal circulation, and into a co-twin in the case of twin–twin transfusion syndrome. Bleeding into the fetus is usually evident on ultrasound examination either because of a vascular malformation such as a sacrococcygeal teratoma or an intracranial arteriovenous malformation, or the presence of an intracranial mass lesion. If a vascular malformation is not present, evaluation for alloimmune thrombocytopenia or other coagulation abnormality should be performed.

Fetomaternal hemorrhage may be preceded by trauma or may be spontaneous. It can be detected through examining for fetal red cells in the maternal circulation (Kleihauer-Betke test) or, more rarely, elevations in maternal serum alpha fetoprotein. MCA Dopplers have been shown to be useful in diagnosing fetal anemia related to fetomaternal hemorrhage.[9] Although fetomaternal hemorrhage is usually self-limited, if hydrops is present, transfusion may prevent demise and has been shown to lead to good neonatal outcomes.[10–13]

Twin–twin transfusion occurs in monochorionic diamniotic twin gestations with unbalanced arteriovenous connections within the placenta. The high-pressure fetal arteries from the donor twin connect with the low-pressure fetal veins from the recipient twin, leading to significant anemia and hypovolemia of the donor. This situation is usually treated through laser ablation of the communicating vessels. MCA Doppler assessment has been shown to be useful in assessing monochorionic diamniotic twins for anemia after 18 weeks.[14] In rare cases of fetal demise of the recipient twin or progressive hydrops after laser therapy, intrauterine transfusion of the donor twin has been described.[15]

Hemoglobinopathies

Hemoglobinopathies can lead to inadequate production or instability of red blood cells in utero. In patients from Asia or the eastern Mediterranean region, homozygous α-thalassemia is one of the most common causes of fetal anemia and hydrops.[16] Unfortunately, because no long-term treatment exists for this condition, fetal transfusion is possible, but it is not usually recommended. Case reports have been published of successful intrauterine therapy, and even using intrauterine transfusion to establish a microchimerism in the neonate, but this is not routine clinical practice.[17,18]

A more rare thalassemia variant $(\gamma\delta\beta)^0$ has also been described in cases of fetal and neonatal anemia. This genetic variation is amenable to in utero therapy, because over time, the unaffected β-globin gene achieves appropriate expression and the affected children then have hematologic phenotypes similar to common β-thalassemia trait.[19]

Glucose-6-phosphate dehydrogenase (G6PD) deficiency is a common X-linked condition in African Americans and persons of Mediterranean descent. This disorder is characterized by hemolytic crises, usually in response to various stimuli, including certain medications (sulfa drugs) and foods (fava beans). Two affected male fetuses developing anemia and hydrops after maternal ingestion of these substances have been reported.[20,21]

Other rare hereditary forms of fetal anemia that have been successfully treated with intrauterine transfusion include xerocytosis and congenital dyserythropoietic anemia.[22,23] In addition, fetal anemia has been caused by Blackfan-Diamond anemia, hemochromatosis, and elliptocytosis.[24,25]

ULTRASOUND FINDINGS

The diagnosis of fetal anemia is made based on clinical suspicion or ultrasound findings. Patients with blood group antibodies on routine prenatal screening are followed serially with antibody titers. For most antibodies, a critical titer of 1:8 to 1:32 (determined by the specific laboratory) is needed to suggest a significant risk of fetal hemolysis and anemia. One exception to this is Kell antibodies, wherein fetal anemia and hydrops have occurred with very low titers.[26] Even with high titers, alloimmunization will not cause fetal anemia if the fetus does not possess the offending antigen. Paternal blood typing should be obtained as long as paternity is certain. If the father of the fetus is heterozygous for the antigen or is not available for testing, the fetus can be tested either through testing free fetal DNA in the maternal circulation or invasive diagnosis with amniocentesis or chorionic villus sampling.

MCA Dopplers

If the fetus is found to be at risk, serial ultrasonographic assessment is recommended. MCA peak velocity measurements have been closely correlated with fetal anemia when corrected for gestational age.[27] The technique requires an adequate transverse view of the sphenoid bone at the base of the skull, and color or power Doppler to visualize the circle of Willis (**Fig. 1**). The MCA vessel closer to the maternal abdominal wall is usually studied, although the posterior vessel can be used if necessary. The angle of insonation with the MCA should be as close to zero as possible, and angle correction should not be used. The Doppler gate should be placed in the proximal MCA, approximately 2 mm from its origin from the circle of Willis. For measurements to be accurate, the fetus must be in a resting state to avoid fetal heart rate accelerations. This factor is of particular concern in the late third trimester when heart rate accelerations are more frequent and false elevations of MCA peak systolic velocity have been reported.[28] Measurements can be initiated at as early as 18 weeks' gestation and should be repeated at 1-week to 4-week intervals based on the results.

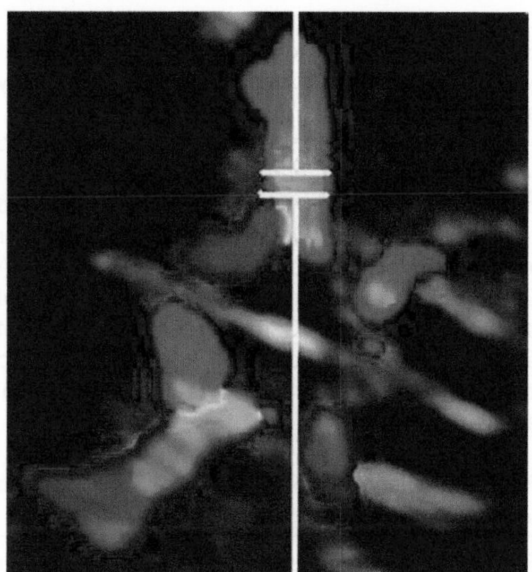

Fig. 1. Correct assessment of the peak systolic velocity of the middle cerebral artery.

A similar strategy is recommended for a fetus suspected of having parvovirus infection from maternal seroconversion during pregnancy. Because the greatest risk for fetal anemia and hydrops occurs during the second trimester, weekly MCA Dopplers are recommended starting at 18 weeks and continuing until 10 to 12 weeks after the initial exposure or known seroconversion to parvovirus.[8]

Assessment of Other Vessels and Structures

Other sonographic approaches to identifying and quantifying fetal anemia have also been attempted. A study looking at placental thickness, extrahepatic and intrahepatic umbilical vein diameters, abdominal circumference, head circumference, head/abdominal circumference ratio, and intraperitoneal volume failed to identify a measurement that could distinguish mild anemia from severe disease.[29] Splenic and liver size were initially promising, but MCA Dopplers were found to have better sensitivity and reproducibility.[30–32]

Cardiac size and function have also been used to predict severe fetal anemia before the onset of hydrops. The cardiofemoral index, calculated using the biventricular outer dimension and femur length, both alone and in combination with MCA Dopplers, has been shown improve detection of severe anemia.[33,34] Cardiac contractility (right and left ventricular shortening fractions) has also been studied but does not accurately predict fetal anemia.[35]

Fetal and Placental Malformations Associated with Anemia

Fetal anemia not caused by alloimmunization or viral infection is usually not suspected until an abnormality is noted on ultrasound performed for another indication. In these cases, a vascular abnormality of the fetus or placenta may be noted or the fetus may have already developed hydrops. Vascular malformations can lead to anemia through "steal" from the regular fetal circulation or internal hemorrhage. These malformations can occur in isolation (intracranial arteriovenous malformations) or as part of another anomaly (sacrococcygeal teratoma).[36] Another malformation is a placental chorioangioma, which also has been associated with fetal anemia and is treatable with intrauterine transfusion.[37]

Hydrops Fetalis

Hydrops fetalis is defined as fluid accumulation in at least 2 of the following fetal compartments: skin, pleural cavity, peritoneal cavity, and pericardial space (**Figs. 2** and **3**).[38] It is also often

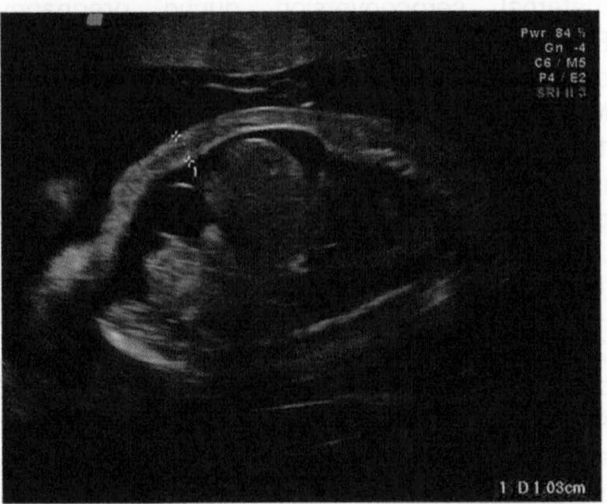

Fig. 2. Fetal hydrops with ascites, pleural effusions, and skin edema.

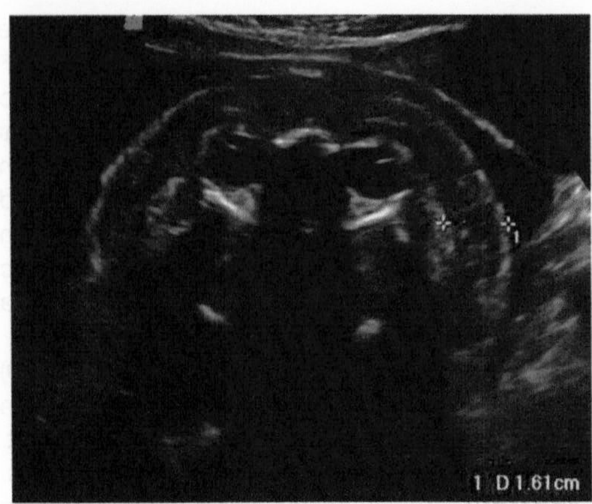

Fig. 3. Marked facial skin edema.

accompanied by polyhydramnios and placentomegaly. Fetal hydrops caused by anemia is a late finding, generally occurring when the hemoglobin has decreased by more than 7 g/dL.[39]

Although hydrops related to fetal anemia is thought to be caused by high-output congestive heart failure, evaluation of ductus venosus flow indicates that hydrops in anemic fetuses may actually precede cardiac decompensation. Anemic hydropic fetuses did not show high central pressure reflected by normal or even low preload index, peak velocity index, and pulsatility index for vein in ductus venosus, despite hyperdynamic circulation or hypervolemia, indicating hydrops fetalis developed before cardiac decompensation.[40]

MANAGEMENT

In addition to ultrasound monitoring for MCA Dopplers and evaluation for hydrops, management of the fetus with anemia involves several possible therapeutic approaches. These modalities have evolved over time and will continue to change with the development of new technologies.

Amniocentesis

The role of invasive procedures in the diagnosis of fetal anemia has changed markedly over the past 50 years. Liley's[4] original description of the assessment of bilirubin in amniotic fluid using absorbance spectrophotometry (delta OD 450) and dividing fetal risk into 3 zones was modified and expanded to the early second trimester by Queenan and colleagues[41] in 1993. This approach, however, was essentially abandoned, because the noninvasive approach with MCA Dopplers has been shown to be superior and has become widely available.[42]

Although amniocentesis still has a role in establishing fetal blood type through DNA testing, assessing for other genetic disorders, and evaluating for congenital viral infection, even this role may be diminishing. New technologies are now available to diagnose fetal blood type from free fetal DNA in the maternal plasma.[43] This approach will allow practitioners to establish fetal blood type without the risk of increasing the degree of sensitization further with an invasive procedure.

Fetal Blood Sampling and Transfusion

Once fetal anemia is suspected by MCA Doppler studies, diagnosis and treatment still relies on determination of fetal hematocrit and the ability to deliver red blood cells to the fetal circulation. With the introduction of improved resolution real-time ultrasound, radiographic-guided intraperitoneal fetal transfusion of the 1960s was replaced by ultrasound-guided intravascular procedures in the 1980s.[44] This approach had the advantage of allowing assessment of the actual fetal hematocrit and enabling immediate fetal access to the oxygen-carrying red blood cells. Intravascular transfusion has been associated with improved survival in both hydropic and nonhydropic fetuses.[45]

Several methods of intravascular fetal access have been described. The most common is the placental insertion of the umbilical vein (video). The intrahepatic portion of the umbilical vein can also be used, and this approach has the advantage of secondary peritoneal absorption of red cells lost into the fetal abdominal cavity.[46] The fetal insertion of the umbilical vein, a free-floating loop of cord, and intracardiac and umbilical artery access are all possible but have been associated with higher rates of complications.

Blood used for fetal transfusion is screened and prepared in the standard fashion, but several additional steps are recommended. Because a fetal type and screen has not usually been performed before transfusion, O-type Rh-negative blood that is also negative for any known alloimmunizing antigens is used. In addition, the blood should be cytomegalovirus-negative, sickle cell–negative, less than 5 days old, gamma-irradiated to reduce the risk of graft versus host reaction, and leukoreduced. The red cells are concentrated to give a final hematocrit of 75% to 85% to minimize the volume that must be transfused.

The volume transfused intravascularly is based on the initial fetal hematocrit and the estimated fetal weight. Several formulas are available that take into account the volume of circulation of the fetus and the placenta. Assuming a combined blood volume of 140 mL/kg of fetal weight, the volume to transfuse can be estimated as

> (the desired increase in hematocrit) × (estimated fetal weight in grams) × (0.14)/(hematocrit of the blood being transfused)

Giannina and colleagues[47] recommend a simple formula of multiplying 0.02 by the estimated fetal weight to obtain the volume of transfused blood to raise the hematocrit by 10%. The target fetal hematocrit is 40% to 50%.

The process of transfusion requires a well-prepared team and notification of both the blood bank and hematology laboratory. Personnel should be assigned the roles of principle operator, ultrasound guidance, assistant for handing syringes and pushing the transfused blood, and assistant for running the fetal sample to the hematology laboratory. Equipment should be prepared on a sterile field, including a sterile sleeve and gel for the ultrasound transducer, a 20-guage needle of appropriate length to reach the target vessel, multiple heparinized 1-mL syringes to obtain fetal samples for hematocrit and other appropriate studies, stopcocks and extension tubing, 10- or 20-mL syringes for transfusing blood, sterile saline to assess adequate needle placement, local anesthetic for the maternal skin, a paralytic agent, and filtered tubing for the blood.

Patients should receive preprocedure intravenous antibiotics to minimize the risk of procedure-related infection, and sedation if needed. For fetuses less than 400 g in whom the transfused volume is usually less than 30 mL, the blood to be transfused is most easily handled by placing into sterile syringes. When larger volumes are transfused, keeping the tubing attached to the blood bank unit and drawing with a stopcock is more efficient.

Once fetal vascular access has been obtained, 0.5 to 1.0 mL of blood is taken to the hematology laboratory to determine the fetal hematocrit, and the fetus is usually paralyzed to prevent fetal movement from dislodging the needle. Vecuronium, 0.1 mg/kg, has replaced pancuronium because it has less effect on the fetal heart rate. If the placental cord insert is used for access, it is necessary to confirm that a fetal vessel has been entered. This placement can be confirmed through evaluating the mean corpuscular volume (MCV) on the sample obtained (>100 is consistent with fetal blood) or injecting saline and watching the turbulence in the cord with color Doppler. If the fetus has already been transfused, the MCV will reflect adult transfused blood and will not be useful. In addition, if the intrahepatic portion of the umbilical vein is accessed, no additional testing is needed to determine if the blood obtained is fetal.

Transfusion is indicated if the fetal hematocrit is 30% or less. Fetal heart rate should be assessed every few minutes during the procedure. Fetal bradycardia can result from too-rapid expansion of the fetal blood volume, hypovolemia from exsanguination caused by streaming, or vasospasm in the umbilical artery. Stopping or slowing the transfusion can lead to resolution in some cases, but if the bradycardia persists, most often the needle should be removed. Cases have been reported of using fetal intravenous epinephrine, 0.1 to 0.3 mg/kg, or volume expansion for in utero resuscitation.[48] If this does not lead to normalization of fetal heart rate, urgent Cesarean delivery is recommended if the fetus is of an appropriate gestational age. For this reason, intrauterine blood sampling and transfusion should be performed on a labor and delivery unit once a fetus is viable.

Fetal Intraperitoneal Transfusion

For fetuses younger than 20 weeks or those in whom fetal and placental positions preclude vascular access, intraperitoneal transfusion can still play a role. In addition, some centers combine intraperitoneal transfusion with the intravascular transfusion, which can result in a more stable fetal hematocrit and a more prolonged interval between procedures.[44]

Complications

In addition to the bradycardia described earlier, other procedure-related complications of intrauterine transfusion include rupture of membranes, preterm labor, intrauterine infection, and fetal demise.[49,50] The incidence of these complications are generally less than 1% (**Table 1**) and have not changed significantly over time, despite the relative decrease in the frequency of intrauterine transfusion. Long-term outcome of fetal anemia and transfusion is reported to be good in 90% to 95% of cases, but an increase in neurodevelopmental impairment is seen.[51]

Other Therapeutic Approaches to Fetal Anemia

Because of the risks and technical difficulties associated with fetal transfusion, immunologic approaches have also been attempted to treat fetal anemia related to alloimmunization. Maternal plasmapheresis and intravenous immunoglobulin (IVIG) therapy have not proven effective in most cases. Two recent reports of fetal peritoneal IVIG therapy seem more promising, but further study is needed.[52,53]

Table 1
Incidence of complications per procedure

Complication	1988–2001	2003–2010
Bradycardia requiring cesarean delivery	2.4%	0.9%
Intrauterine infection	0.3%	0%
Rupture of membranes	0.1%	0%
Fetal death	0.9%	0.9%

Data from Van Kamp IL, Klumper FJ, Oepkes D, et al. Complications of intrauterine intravascular transfusion for fetal anemia due to maternal red-cell alloimmunization. Am J Obstet Gynecol 2005;192:171–7; and Johnstone-Ayliffe C, Prior T, Ong C, et al. Early procedure-related complications of fetal blood sampling and intrauterine transfusion for fetal anemia. Acta Obstet Gynecol Scand 2011;91:458–62.

Other adjuvant therapies that improve fetal outcome are antenatal steroids after viability and oral maternal phenobarbital therapy, 30 mg 3 times daily for 7 to 10 days, after the last intrauterine transfusion. Phenobarbital enhances fetal hepatic maturity and has been shown to significantly decrease the need for neonatal exchange transfusions in cases of alloimmunization.[54,55]

DELIVERY PLANNING

For fetal anemia requiring transfusion, delivery is usually recommended between 34 and 38 weeks, with the timing based on the last transfusion. The risks of intrauterine transfusion generally outweigh the benefits by 35 weeks. For fetal anemia managed conservatively, delivery is recommended at 38 weeks in the presence of ongoing risk (alloimmunization or chronic fetomaternal hemorrhage). The role of amniotic fluid testing for fetal lung maturity is limited, because delaying delivery until maturity is documented if another transfusion would be required is not recommended.

Because of the high risk of neonatal anemia and hyperbilirubinemia in patients with alloimmunization, communication with the pediatric team and aggressive neonatal monitoring are recommended. Infants should be followed for neurologic development and hearing assessment, because high bilirubin levels have been associated with hearing loss.

PEARLS AND PITFALLS

Several pearls and pitfalls should be considered when caring for patients with fetal anemia. Although MCA Dopplers can provide excellent

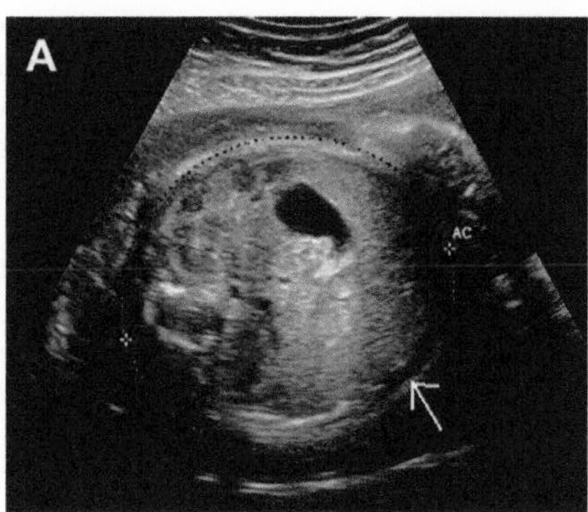

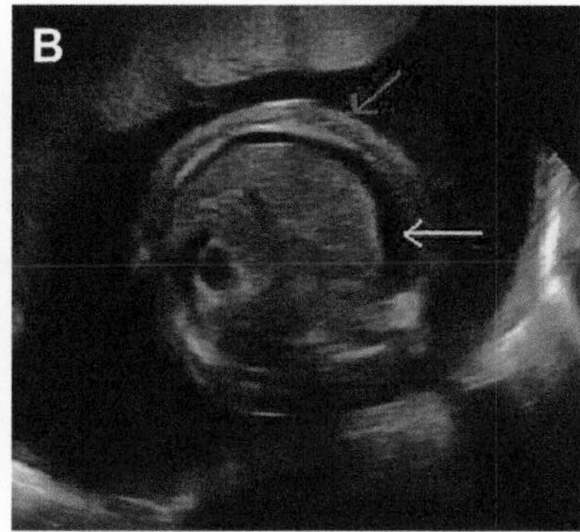

Fig. 4. (*A*) Fetal fat (*white arrow*), which can look like ascites or skin edema. (*B*) True hydrops with skin edema (*red arrow*) and ascites (*yellow arrow*).

information regarding the presence of severe fetal anemia, the technique is known to miss milder forms of anemia. In addition, if a zero angle of insonance cannot be achieved because of fetal position, the peak systolic velocity may be falsely lowered. Finally, MCA Dopplers have been noted to be falsely elevated after 35 weeks, and therefore alternate approaches to patients in the late third trimester should be used.[54]

Another potential pitfall is sonographic diagnosis of fetal hydrops based on fetal fat rather than skin edema or ascites (**Fig. 4**). This situation can be avoided by taking into account coronal views to look for ascites, and other fetal measurements to look for markers of fetal macrosomia.

A potential pitfall when performing fetal blood sampling is accessing a maternal vascular space rather than a fetal umbilical vein at the placental insertion. MCV measurements on blood sample and assessing turbulence in the cord with instillation of saline can identify this situation.

SUMMARY

Fetal anemia is a treatable cause of hydrops fetalis and can be caused by several different clinical situations. Management of fetal anemia relies on appropriate suspicion based on clinical history or sonographic findings, application of both invasive and noninvasive diagnostic technologies, and a combination of in utero therapy, delivery planning, and postnatal management. MCA Doppler velocimetry can predict significant fetal anemia accurately before 35 weeks' gestation. Intrauterine transfusion can successfully treat fetal anemia from a variety of causes. In general, in utero treatment of fetal anemia, particularly before the onset of hydrops, leads to good neonatal and childhood outcome.

SUPPLEMENTARY DATA

Video related to this article can be found online at doi:10.1016/j.cult.2012.08.009.

REFERENCES

1. Bowman JM. RhD hemolytic disease of the newborn. N Engl J Med 1998;339:1775–7.
2. Ballantyne JW. Remarks on Sclerema & OEdema Neonatorum. Br Med J 1890;1:403–6.
3. Levine P, Stetson R. An usual case of intragroup agglutination. JAMA 1939;113:126–7.
4. Liley AW. Liquor amnii analysis in the management of pregnancy complicated by rhesus sensitization. Am J Obstet Gynecol 1961;82:1359–70.
5. Liley AW. Intrauterine transfusion of foetus in haemolytic disease. BMJ 1963;2:1107–9.
6. Moise KJ. Fetal anemia due to non-Rhesus-D red-cell alloimmunization. Semin Fetal Neonatal Med 2008;13:207e–14e.
7. Rimon E, Peltz R, Gamzu R, et al. Management of Kell isoimmunization – evaluation of a Doppler-guided approach. Ultrasound Obstet Gynecol 2006;28:814–20.
8. Lamont RF, Sobel JD, Vaisbuch E, et al. Parvovirus B19 infection in human pregnancy. BJOG 2011;118:175–86.
9. Cosmi E, Rampon M, Saccardi C, et al. Middle cerebral artery peak systolic velocity in the diagnosis of fetomaternal hemorrhage. Int J Gynaecol Obstet 2012;117:128–30.
10. Rubod C, Houfflin V, Belot F, et al. Successful in utero treatment of chronic and massive fetomaternal hemorrhage with fetal hydrops. Fetal Diagn Ther 2006;21:410–3.
11. Cardwell MS. Successful treatment of hydrops fetalis caused by fetomaternal hemorrhage: a case report. Am J Obstet Gynecol 1988;158:131–2.

12. Rouse D, Weiner C. Ongoing fetomaternal hemorrhage treated by serial fetal intravascular transfusions. Obstet Gynecol 1990;76:974–5.
13. Thorp JA, Cohen GR, Yeast JD, et al. Nonimmune hydrops caused by massive fetomaternal hemorrhage and treated by intravascular transfusion. Am J Perinatol 1992;9:22–4.
14. Klaritsch P, Deprest J, Van Mieghem T, et al. Reference ranges for middle cerebral artery peak systolic velocity in monochorionic diamniotic twins: a longitudinal study. Ultrasound Obstet Gynecol 2009;34:149–54.
15. Ozcan T, Thornburg L, Mingione M, et al. Use of middle cerebral artery peak systolic velocity and intrauterine transfusion for management of twin-twin transfusion and single fetal intrauterine demise. J Matern Fetal Neonatal Med 2006;19:807–9.
16. Nakayama R, Yamada D, Steinmiller V, et al. Hydrops fetalis secondary to Bart hemoglobinopathy. Obstet Gynecol 1986;67:176–80.
17. Ng PC, Fok TF, Lee CH, et al. Is homozygous alpha-thalassaemia a lethal condition in the 1990s? Acta Paediatr 1998;87:1197–9.
18. Hayward A, Ambruso D, Battaglia F, et al. Microchimerism and tolerance following intrauterine transplantation and transfusion for alpha-thalassemia-1. Fetal Diagn Ther 1998;13:8–14.
19. Verhovsek M, Shah NR, Wilcox I, et al. Severe fetal and neonatal hemolytic anemia due to a 198 kb deletion removing the complete β-globin gene cluster. Pediatr Blood Cancer 2012;59:941–4.
20. Perkins RP. Hydrops fetalis and stillbirth in a male glucose-6-phosphate dehydrogenase-deficient fetus possibly due to maternal ingestion of sulfisoxazole. Am J Obstet Gynecol 1971;3:379–81.
21. Mentzer WC, Collier E. Hydrops fetalis associated with erythrocyte G-6-PD deficiency and maternal ingestion of fava beans and ascorbic acid. J Pediatr 1975;86:565–7.
22. Ogburn PL Jr, Ramin KD, Danilenko-Dixon D, et al. In utero erythrocyte transfusion for fetal xerocytosis associated with severe anemia and non-immune hydrops fetalis. Am J Obstet Gynecol 2001;185:238–9.
23. Remacha AF, Badell I, Pujol-Moix N, et al. Hydrops fetalis-associated congenital dyserythropoietic anemia treated with intrauterine transfusions and bone marrow transplantation. Blood 2002;100:356–8.
24. Amann C, Geipel A, Müller A, et al. Fetal anemia of unknown cause–a diagnostic challenge. Ultraschall Med 2011;32(Suppl 2):E134–140.
25. Zhang EG, Regan F, Layton M, et al. Managing the difficult case of fetal anemia. J Matern Fetal Neonatal Med 2011;24(12):1498–503.
26. Bowman JM, Pollock JM, Manning FA, et al. Maternal Kell blood group alloimmunization. Obstet Gynecol 1992;79:239–44.
27. Mari G, Deter RL, Carpenter RL, et al. Noninvasive diagnosis by Doppler ultrasonography of fetal anemia due to maternal red-cell alloimmunization. Collaborative Group for Doppler assessment of the blood velocity in anemic fetuses. N Engl J Med 2000;342:9–14.
28. Zimmerman R, Carpenter RJ Jr, Durig P, et al. Longitudinal measurement of peak systolic velocity in the fetal middle cerebral artery for monitoring pregnancies complicated by red cell alloimmunisation: a prospective multicenter trial with intention-to-treat. BJOG 2002;109:746–52.
29. Nicolaides KH, Fontanarosa M, Gabbe SG, et al. Failure of ultrasonographic parameters to predict the severity of fetal anemia in rhesus isoimmunization. Am J Obstet Gynecol 1988;158:920.
30. Bahado-Singh R, Oz U, Mari G, et al. Fetal splenic size in anemia due to Rh-alloimmunization. Obstet Gynecol 1998;92:828–32.
31. Roberts AB, Mitchell JM, Lake Y, et al. Ultrasonographic surveillance in red blood cell alloimmunization. Am J Obstet Gynecol 2001;184:1251–5.
32. Dukler D, Oepkes D, Seaward G, et al. Noninvasive tests to predict fetal anemia: a study comparing Doppler and ultrasound parameters. Am J Obstet Gynecol 2003;188:1310–4.
33. Cabral ACV, Reis ZSN, Leite HV, et al. Cardiofemoral index as an ultrasound marker of fetal anemia in isoimmunized pregnancy. Int J Gynaecol Obstet 2008;100:60–4.
34. Cabral ACV, Reis ZSN, Apocalypse IG, et al. Combined use of the cardiofemoral index and middle cerebral artery Doppler velocimetry for the prediction of fetal anemia. Int J Gynaecol Obstet 2010;111:205–8.
35. Sikkel E, Klumper FJ, Oepkes D, et al. Fetal cardiac contractility before and after intrauterine transfusion. Ultrasound Obstet Gynecol 2005;26:611–7.
36. Yamaguchi Y, Tsukimori K, Hojo S, et al. Spontaneous rupture of sacrococcygeal teratoma associated with acute fetal anemia. Ultrasound Obstet Gynecol 2006;28:720–2.
37. Hamill N, Rijhsinghani A, Williamson RA, et al. Prenatal diagnosis and management of fetal anemia secondary to a large chorioangioma. Obstet Gynecol 2003;102:1185–8.
38. Platt LD, DeVore GR. In utero diagnosis of hydrops fetalis: ultrasound methods. Clin Perinatol 1982;9:627–36.
39. Nicolaides KH, Thilaganathan B, Rodeck CH, et al. Erythroblastosis and reticulocytosis in anemic fetuses. Am J Obstet Gynecol 1988;159:1063–5.
40. Tongsong T, Tongprasert F, Srisupundit K, et al. Venous Doppler studies in low-output and high-output hydrops fetalis. Am J Obstet Gynecol 2010;203:488.e1–6.
41. Queenan JT, Tomai TP, Ural SH, et al. Deviation in amniotic fluid optical density at a wavelength of 450 nm in Rh-immunized pregnancies from 14 to

40 weeks' gestation: a proposal for clinical management. Am J Obstet Gynecol 1993;168:1370–6.
42. Oepkes D, Seaward PG, Vandenbussche FP, et al. Doppler ultrasonography versus amniocentesis to predict fetal anemia. N Engl J Med 2006;355:156–64.
43. Cardo L, García BP, Alvarez FV. Non-invasive fetal RHD genotyping in the first trimester of pregnancy. Clin Chem Lab Med 2010;48:1121–6.
44. Moise KJ. Management of rhesus alloimmunization in pregnancy. Obstet Gynecol 2008;112:164–76.
45. Harman CR, Bowman JM, Manning FA, et al. Intrauterine transfusion–intraperitoneal versus intravascular approach: a case-control comparison. Am J Obstet Gynecol 1990;162:1053–9.
46. Nicolini U, Santolaya J, Ojo OE, et al. The fetal intrahepatic umbilical vein as an alternative to cord needling for prenatal diagnosis and therapy. Prenat Diagn 1988;8:665–71.
47. Giannina G, Moise KJ, Dorman K. A simple method to estimate the volume for fetal intravascular transfusion. Fetal Diagn Ther 1998;13:94–7.
48. Shalev E, Peleg D. Fetal cardiac resuscitation. Lancet 1993;341:305–6.
49. Van Kamp IL, Klumper FJ, Oepkes D, et al. Complications of intrauterine intravascular transfusion for fetal anemia due to maternal red-cell alloimmunization. Am J Obstet Gynecol 2005;192:171–7.
50. Johnstone-Ayliffe C, Prior T, Ong C, et al. Early procedure-related complications of fetal blood sampling and intrauterine transfusion for fetal anemia. Acta Obstet Gynecol Scand 2011;91:458–62.
51. Lindenburg IT, Smits-Wintjens VE, van Klink JM, et al. On behalf of the LOTUS study group. Long-term neurodevelopmental outcome after intrauterine transfusion for hemolytic disease of the fetus/newborn: the LOTUS study. Am J Obstet Gynecol 2012;206:141.e1–8.
52. Matsuda H, Yoshida M, Wakamatsu H, et al. Fetal intraperitoneal injection of immunoglobulin diminishes alloimmune hemolysis. J Perinatol 2011;31:289–92.
53. Yoshida M, Matsuda H, Hayata E, et al. Successful treatment of fetal intraperitoneal administration of immunoglobulin in a case of fetal hemolytic anemia with 131,072-fold anti-E alloimmunization. Case Rep Obstet Gynecol 2011;2011:157510.
54. Trevett TN, Dorman K, Lamvu G, et al. Antenatal maternal administration of phenobarbital for the prevention of exchange transfusion in neonates with hemolytic disease of the fetus and newborn. Am J Obstet Gynecol 2005;192:478–82.
55. Mari G. Middle cerebral artery peak systolic velocity for the diagnosis of fetal anemia: the untold story. Ultrasound Obstet Gynecol 2005;25:323–30.

Training for Ultrasound Procedures

Loralei L. Thornburg, MD

KEYWORDS

• Ultrasound procedures • Amniocentesis training • Chorionic villus sampling training • Fetal blood sampling training • Cordocentesis training • Fellowship training • Simulation

KEY POINTS

- All procedures performed in pregnancy carry risk, and therefore the clinician must understand the risks and benefits before engaging in any procedure.
- Simulation, team development, and planning can help to minimize the risks of procedural complications.
- Multiple simulation methods exist for these procedures, although outcome data are limited.

Videos on amniocentesis approach, term amniocentesis, transabdominal CVS, and transcervical CVS accompany this article.

INTRODUCTION

Ultrasound provides a window in the intrauterine environment, which makes the ability to intervene, assess, and provide fetal therapy during pregnancy a possibility. Ultrasound is used to guide several procedures in pregnancy, including amniocentesis, chorionic villus sampling (CVS), fetal blood sampling (FBS), fetal biopsy, and dilation and curettage. In addition, ultrasound is sometimes used as a compliment to fetal surgery for cardiac monitoring. This article focuses on the training for the most common ultrasound-guided procedures of amniocentesis, FBS, and CVS. Training for ultrasound procedures has considerable variability in the approach and methodologies used.

DIDACTIC KNOWLEDGE AND PROCEDURE PREPARATION

Training for any procedure must include some combination of didactic training, observation, simulation, and performance in a monitored setting. Procedural training and training competent physicians has become an area of intensive research interest across the surgical disciplines. There are several significant threats to the traditional apprenticeship method of training, including a decreasing number of procedures, increased numbers of trainees, and work hour limitations.[1] As noted by Tafra[2] in a discussion on training for ultrasound-based biopsy, "It is frightening to speculate the level of mortality that might ensue if pilots received the same level of training that surgeons are currently subjected to in learning new surgical procedures." In no other specialty is this more important than in obstetrics, because not 1 but 2 patients are at risk.

Before any procedure, the trainee must understand the reasons, alternatives, complications, and follow-up for any procedure performed. The trainee should also understand how the test will be used to guide clinical care, and follow-up testing that may be offered, as well as how this will determine further care during pregnancy. Testing that does not change management or improve outcomes should be avoided, and therefore the

Disclosures: None.
Conflicts of interest: None.
Division of Maternal Fetal Medicine, Department of OB/GYN, University of Rochester Medical Center, University of Rochester, 601 Elmwood Avenue, Box 668, Rochester, NY 14642, USA
E-mail address: loralei_thornburg@urmc.rochester.edu

Ultrasound Clin 8 (2013) 89–103
http://dx.doi.org/10.1016/j.cult.2012.08.017
1556-858X/13/$ – see front matter

trainee should be able to iterate how this testing will be used and the implications of the possible different results. Data are clear that those who perform fewer procedures have higher complication rates, and, therefore, only those physicians who are comfortable and well trained should attempt any ultrasound-based procedure.[3]

Web-based didactics followed by simulation seem to be as effective as traditional didactic lectures with simulation and may be a valuable way to provide education for fellows spread over multiple sites or years.[4] For simple procedures, summary feedback (feedback after completing a task) and continuous feedback (feedback while performing a skill) are equally affective in the development of learner skills.[5] Therefore, clinicians can safely provide educational feedback after completion when performing procedures that occur while the patient is awake. Training must be spread over time to have the best retention and allow the trainee to successfully transfer skills to different clinical situations.[6] The clinician educator must also understand the complexity and tension of education with safety, and there is a complex dynamic of maintaining control while allowing trainee independence.[7] In addition, the teacher must be able to move between a more reserved, nonintervention approach when trainees are within their safety zones, and a more mindful, thoughtful approach with a more complex portion of the case or if complications arise, a phenomenon known in the surgical literature as slowing down when you should.[8,9]

PROCEDURE PLANNING: TEAM DEVELOPMENT

Regardless of the procedure involved, safe performance requires a systematic approach (**Box 1**). The patient must be appropriately counseled and must consent to the procedure. In addition, the provider must be certain about the tests that need to be performed and the laboratory requirements to perform these tests. The amount, type, and preparation of the samples should be clearly delineated. For those tests that are performed rarely or are being sent for outside testing, the provider, genetic counselor, and sonographer should have a team huddle before any procedure to ensure that the appropriate specimens are obtained and that they are handled and processed in the appropriate way. In addition, if there are any planned administrations, such as blood products or medications, or if these may be needed, the provider and any assistants should be sure that these are present and properly prepared and labeled if drawn out of the original containers.

Box 1
Planning for procedures

1. Consents and requisitions needed are present, signed, and completely filled out
2. Any labels or transport materials needed are present
3. Necessary equipment present (duplicates, extras easily available)
4. Team aware of planned procedure, methods to be used
5. Team aware of how extra equipment will be called for or obtained
6. Any solutions, medications, or blood products needed are present, labeled, and expirations confirmed
7. Dosages are confirmed, or dosage charts available
8. If samples will be taken for testing during the procedure, the team is aware of who will obtain sample, who will evaluate the sample, and the laboratory is aware of timing and is prepared to receive sample
9. Extra personnel are available in case complications arise, and are aware that the procedure is occurring

Extra and duplicate equipment should be easily available in case something becomes contaminated or the procedure or approach changes during the performance.

For more complex procedures, such as FBS, in which multiple samples and staff are needed, results have be obtained rapidly, and multiple medications are administered, a checklist and specific roles for each team member should be developed. Simulation of these events can help to find any systematic problems, and staff preprocedure huddles can ensure that all members of the team have completed their tasks and are fully prepared and aware of the plan. Simulation of the team approach has not been studied in fetal procedures; however, it has been shown to improve performance in other complex, team-based procedures.[10]

A standard approach to the procedure, either as a formalized time-out or a routine list of questions that is done before all procedures, can help to eliminate errors. At a minimum, the attending physician should confirm the patient (and ideally have the patient confirm the spelling and identifiers to be used on the sample), the procedure, the indication and tests being performed, the presence of consent, any allergies (especially latex or iodine if these are going to be used in preparation of the skin), and the patient's blood type. The patient should be present for this, and should confirm the information. Creation of standardized checklists (**Box 2**) for each step to be performed, in order, and standardized among teams, has been shown to reduce complications with other complex, invasive medical procedures such as central lines.[11] These measures can be especially helpful for the trainee, because they allow a structured approach, as well as empowering the sonologist or other personnel to recognize and point out a deviation from the planned approach.[11]

PLANNING THE APPROACH

Providers generally perform ultrasound-guided procedures in 1 of 2 ways: either the provider performs the procedure with guidance from a sonologist, or providers use a 2-handed technique and guide for themselves. Regardless, providers should perform at least a brief assessment of the intrauterine environment themselves and ensure that they are confident in the planned approach. The provider should also perform an assessment for any likely pitfalls, such as the presence of leiomyomata, location of the placenta, and uterine and fetal positions, such that if the situation changes after beginning the procedure, they are able to rapidly change their approach. For patients with significant abdominal adiposity, the provider or sonologist should assess the distance from the skin to the target by ultrasound and ensure that a needle of an adequate length is chosen (**Fig. 1**).

Box 2
Example of a procedure checklist

Amniocentesis for singleton with guiding sonologist:

1. Consent present, signed
2. Materials verified
3. Patient, procedure, amount of fluid needed confirmed
4. Labels confirmed, including spelling, date
5. Patient's blood type and allergies confirmed
6. Patient positioned, draped to protect clothing
7. Physician locates site, explains approach to sonologist/patient
8. Skin marked
9. Equipment, needle, syringes checked and confirmed correct
10. Prep of skin performed
11. Pocket reconfirmed by sonologist
12. Simulation of procedure by physician using needle guide or finger to reconfirm approach
13. Procedure performed by physician, sonologist guiding
14. Initial fluid discarded
15. Sample withdrawn under direct guidance
16. Fetal heart rate/wellbeing reconfirmed
17. Sample labeled, prepared for transportation
18. Postprocedure counseling of patient
19. Requisitions and samples appropriately handed off to laboratory

In addition, the team should discuss the approach and have an understanding of the terminology that will be used during any guidance. For example, a directive of "Toward me" from the guiding operator would be interpreted by most as a suggested correction of moving the tip of the needle or catheter toward the guiding operator (generally on the right side of the patient) by moving the hub away, but it could be misinterpreted by the trainee to mean the hub of the needle, which would move the tip away from the desired field. A preprocedure discussion of how much movement is appropriate, directionality, as well as a discussion of approach while performing the preprocedure planning ultrasound can help to eliminate any confusion.

APPROACHES TO LEARNING: PROCEDURE SIMULATION

Simulation of procedures can be helpful to aid in trainee comfort with procedures before attempting the procedure in situ. In addition, the use of simulators can improve the trainee's understanding of the

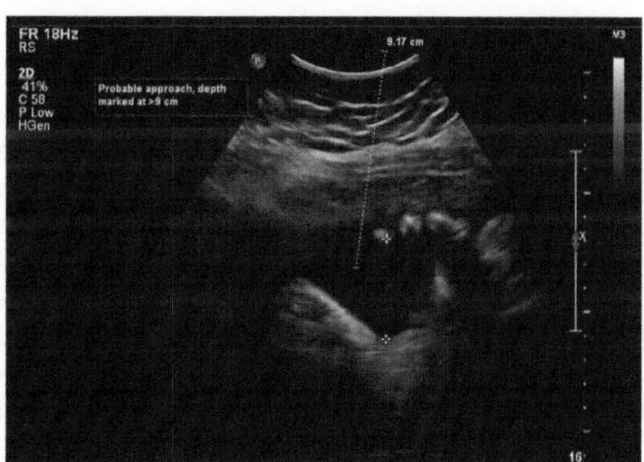

Fig. 1. Marking the depth by ultrasound in the probable plane and direction of approach can ensure that an appropriate needle length is chosen. Note the line depicting depth from above the skin to the target pocket of amniotic fluid.

approach and the viewing of the needle/catheter by the ultrasound. Simple simulators for a variety of procedures exist, including commercially available simulators as well as more homemade simulators, such as gelatin suspensions, fetal pigs, cow hearts, balloons within zippered storage bags, fresh placenta, and olives within chicken breasts.[12–17] These have been shown to improve trainee comfort with the procedure approaches, and speed with completion of procedures, but clinical outcomes related to simulation training with these methods are limited.[16]

Simulation can also be done by performing procedures on noncontinuing pregnancies. Because the pregnancy is going to be interrupted, these can represent a natural opportunity to practice those procedures that carry a risk of disrupting a desired pregnancy. Depending on the gestational age of the pregnancy, procedure training options can include CVS, amniocentesis, and/or FBS. These procedures can either be purely educational or can be used to provide samples for clinical use in a situation in which the risks of pregnancy interruption are not a concern. Examples of this include amniocentesis before induction for fetal demise to improve chromosome yield for genetic testing, or if the termination is being done for fetal anomalies or genetic risk. Because the patient is often anesthetized or sedated, the teaching provider is able to provide more direct guidance and feedback than with an awake patient. Although patients might be expected to be poorly tolerant of this, at our institution 40% of those approached agree, without clear variation between demographic groups.[18] The data suggest that this training did not interfere with operating room timing of procedures, increasing the length of the case by only an average of 9 minutes.[19] CVS was first perfected as a technique in phase 2 and 3 trials on terminating pregnancies.[20]

PROCEDURE-SPECIFIC CONCERNS

Amniocentesis

Amniocentesis provides a method of access to the fetal amniotic fluid. The most common indication is the assessment of fetal genetic information in the setting of fetal anomalies, advanced maternal age, or increased screening risk. However, amniocentesis can also be used to diagnose ruptured membranes or chorioamnionitis, to instill medications into the amniotic cavity, and to assess fetal lung maturity. Risks include failed procedures, chorioamnionitis, fetal injury, preterm premature rupture of membranes, preterm birth, and miscarriage.

Although amniocentesis was first done without the use of ultrasound guidance, it has now become a strictly ultrasound-based procedure. Ultrasound guidance has been shown to substantially increase the safety with this procedure, as well as to decrease the risk of multiple insertions, bloody samples, failed procedures, and trauma.[21] In addition, operator experience is associated with better success and fewer complications, with those physicians performing more than 50 procedures having a higher single-pass success rate than those with fewer than 50 procedures.[22,23]

Initial complications rates quoted for amniocentesis were at least 2%,[24] with higher risks with early amniocentesis.[25] More recent estimates range between 0.6% and 1% (confidence interval 0.19%–1.52%), and transplacental passage does not seem to increase these risks.[26,27] The First and Second-Trimester Evaluation of Risk for Aneuploidy trial reported rates of complications after amniocentesis as low as 0.06%,[28] although this has been called into question.[23,27] In part because of these low risks, the American College of Obstetrics and Gynecology now recommends that all women, regardless of age, have access to screening, as well as invasive procedures if desired.[29] Loss rates are not increased with up to 2 attempts in a single visit so, if a trainee fails to obtain fluid, the supervising physician can perform the procedure without increasing the risks to the pregnancy.[26]

As with any procedure, training for amniocentesis must include some combination of didactic training, observation, simulation, and performance in a monitored setting. For those patients undergoing amniocentesis for genetic testing before induction of labor with a fetal demise, this can be an ideal opportunity to allow a trainee to perform the amniocentesis, because the risks of miscarriage, preterm birth, membrane rupture, or fetal injury are no longer a concern. In addition, those amniocenteses that are performed for fetal lung maturity, in which the risks of prematurity are substantially lower, or those for amnioreduction, either in cases of extreme polyhydramnios or as a therapy for twin-twin transfusion, in which the pockets are often large, fundal, and easily accessible, can provide excellent training opportunities. However, these procedures still carry risks and the trainee should have had appropriate preparation, as with any procedure.

As with all procedures, all members of the team should be aware of their roles and the tests/procedures that will be performed. Providers generally perform amniocentesis procedures in 1 of 2 ways. Either the providers perform the procedure with guidance from a sonologist or use a 2-handed technique and guide for themselves. Some providers also perform amniocentesis using a needle guide, which allows passage of the needle directly in line with the probe. Although this has the advantage of advancing the needle in line with the ultrasound beam, it makes readjustment more difficult, because the probe cannot be moved without moving the needle in older models; therefore, if the fetus moves or the pocket changes, the direction of the needle cannot be easily readjusted. This limitation is less of a concern with newer needle guides, which allow removal of the needle after entry.[30] These guides may be helpful for cases of severe oligohydramnios, because the needle entry point and path are more easily predetermined.[26] There are minimal data regarding which approach is the safest, and providers should perform the procedure in the way with which they are most comfortable.[3]

If providers are going to have a sonologist perform the guidance, the sonologist should ensure that they are aware of the approach, and the method that the provider will be using. If the sonologist has limited guiding experience, then having a more senior member of the staff available to step in or provide aid can be helpful. The approach should be visualized both by ultrasound (ie, having the probe show the approach that will be used by the needle) and then with the view adjusted to show how the ultrasound beam will view the approaching needle. The provider should indent the uterus under ultrasound visualization to ensure that the directionality and view by ultrasound are correct before preparing the skin (**Fig. 2**, Videos 1 and 2). The plastic sheath from a needle can be ideal to mimic the needle pressure and direction for the trainee, and also leaves a small circle on the skin and provides a guiding mark for the prep (**Fig. 3**). This is a nonmarking, nonpainful way of quickly simulating the procedure before starting. As an alternative, marking with a surgical marker can also be done.

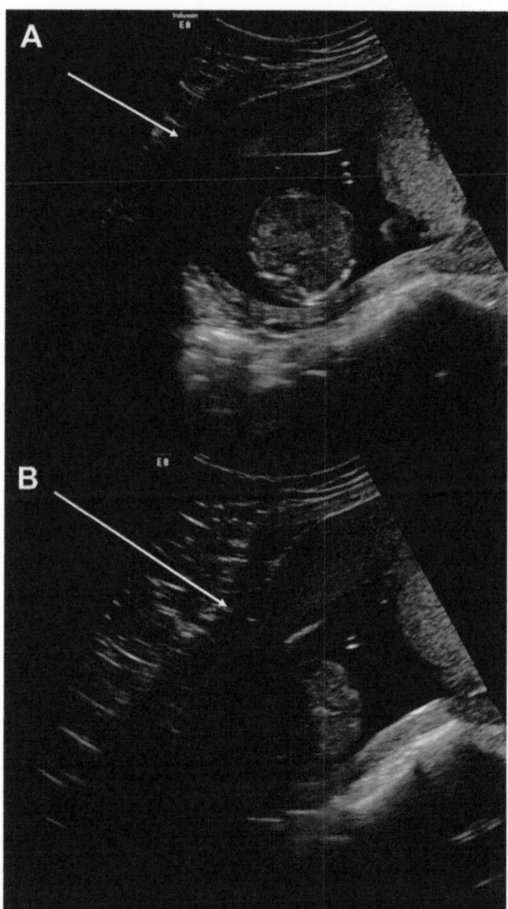

Fig. 2. Planning the ultrasound approach. The provider should indent the uterus while watching under ultrasound guidance to get a sense of the direction, path, and pressure needed, as well as to ensure appropriate orientation of the transducer before prepping the skin. Note the location and contour difference in the uterine wall (*arrows*) between (*A*) and (*B*) as it is distorted by gentle surface pressure from a single finger. This is the time to check with the sonographer about the plan, approach, and desired insonation angle for visualization.

AMNIOCENTESIS SIMULATION

For amniocentesis, simulation seems to improve adherence to procedural checklists from 55% to 95% after training, as well as improving global assessment of skills.[31] Multiple simulators for amniocentesis exist, and these are probably the easiest procedures to create homemade simulators for, including gelatin suspensions, fetal pigs, and balloons within zippered storage bags.[13–15,32] Gelatin simulators (balloons or objects suspended in a gelatin mold) have the advantage of using cheap, readily available materials and not involving any fixed animal tissues, making their storage easy, with good learner feedback (**Fig. 4**A).[14] However, these simulators have the disadvantage of leaving a track within the gelatin, which causes noise and scatter with the model in repeated uses, requiring the gelatin to be reheated and remolded.[15] In addition, there is no fetus to avoid, and the targets are small, which limits the need for the learner to find an approach.[15] Other gelatin models have been used with more complex layering, targets, and membranes (see **Fig. 4**B), but there is still ghosting within the gelatin, which is particularly problematic if the needle markedly changes direction during the procedure leaving a fan-like ghosting plane behind. These problems limit the ability to reuse the model without repair/replacement.[13] In addition, a water bath within a container with a limited opening

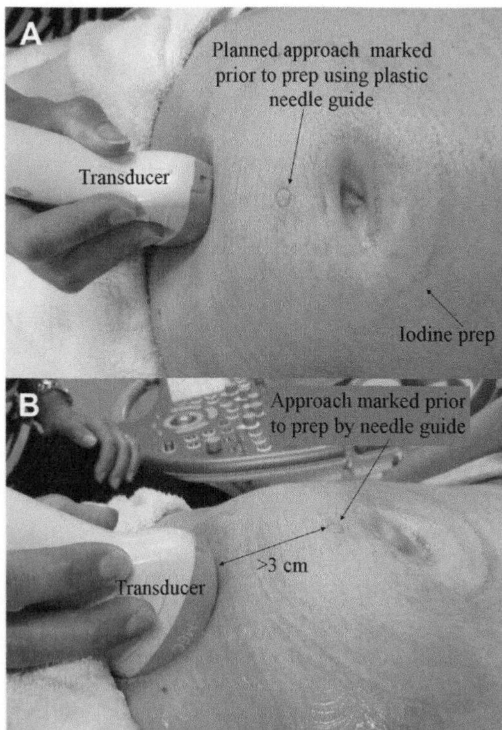

Fig. 3. Prepped abdomen with visible mark from needle cover (*A*) that persists after prepping. When training for amniocentesis, a needle cover can be used to determine the direction and approach under ultrasound guidance as well as to mark the needle entry site. This technique provides a quick, in situ simulation for the trainee; allows the attending physician to see and correct the planned approach, if needed; and provides a visual cue on the abdomen for the site location. Note how the transducer is placed more than 3 cm from the chosen needle site (*B*), allowing visualization of needle approach because the sound beam can be angled up using the natural contour of the maternal abdomen.

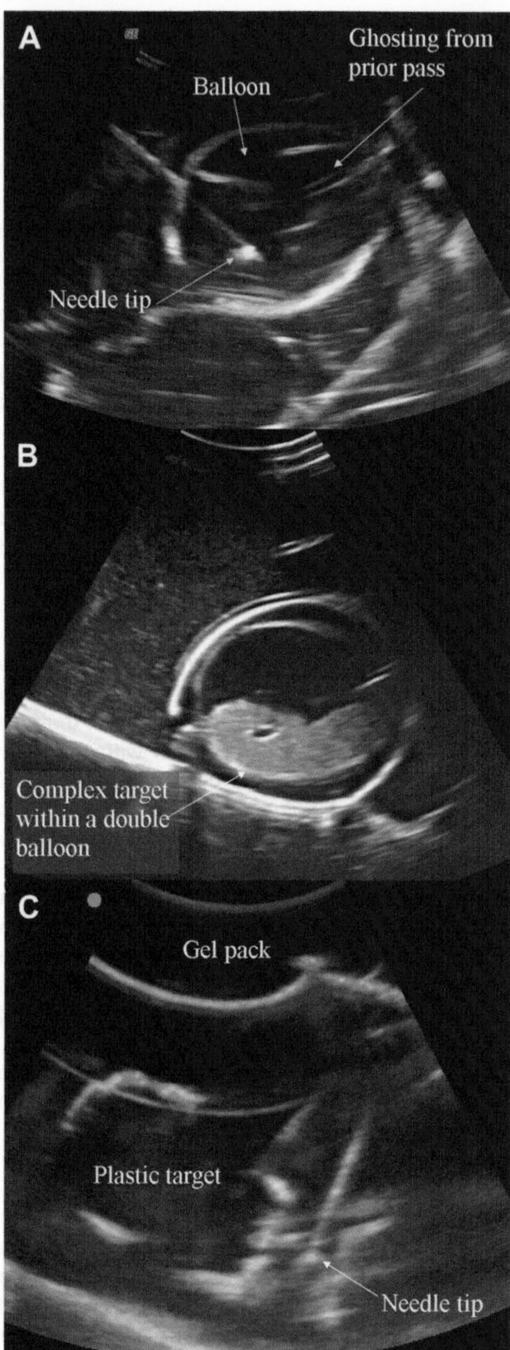

Fig. 4. Simple simulators for amniocentesis training. Images obtained using various gelatin simulators to simulate amniocentesis approach. The targets can be simple (*A*), such as suspended water balloon, or complex (*B*) with multiple balloons containing objects or fluids of different densities. Note the ghosting of prior passes within the simulator. A simple water bath with objects within it and a gel pack suspended above also results in reasonable images (*C*).

(for example, a polystyrene cooler with a hole cut in the lid) can also be used. An object can be suspended within the fluid, a gelatin pack placed over opening, and then ultrasound used to guide procedures performed through this window (see **Fig. 4**C).

Others have used fetal pigs in utero for models.[15] These provide a more realistic pocket, a fetus that must be avoided, and more realistic overall look to the procedure (**Fig. 5**).[15] They do not show needle tracks, and can be used for large numbers of procedures without needing replacement. They can also be used to simulate in utero thoracic or bladder shunt placement.[32] However, they are slightly more expensive for initial setup, but, because of their usefulness over a larger number of procedures without repair, they may be less expensive on a per procedure/per learner

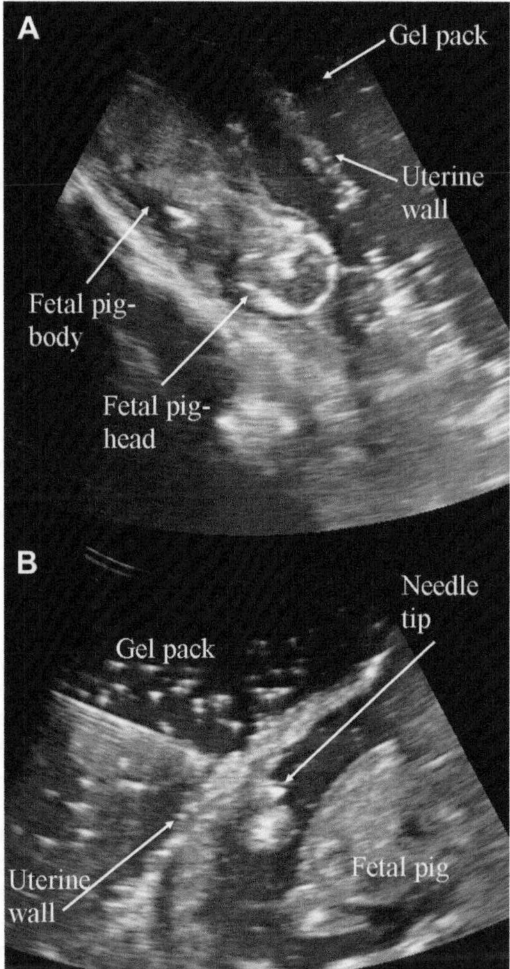

Fig. 5. Fixed fetal pig used for amniocentesis training. The images are realistic when using a fixed fetal pig (*A*) within a fixed and fluid-filled pig uterus to simulate an amniocentesis approach (*B*).

basis. They require some management and handling of biologic specimens, and there are learners who have objections to the use of animal models. There are commercially available amniocentesis or combination amniocentesis/FBS simulators as well; however, again, the expense limits use for many in teaching practice.[33,34]

Regardless of the method, simulation of amniocentesis seems to be associated with a steeper learning curve to achieve excellence. In addition, it seems that simulation with direct, real-time feedback mechanism may improve the learning curve.[35] In the work by Nizard and colleagues,[35] the use of electronic guidance systems improved the speed at which learners achieved competence, defined as ability to visualize the needle throughout the pass, although all learners were able to do this by completion of 75 to 100 procedures regardless of simulation method. The greatest improvement was in the midpoint of the learning curve, procedures 25 to 75, underscoring the importance of ongoing direct observation and feedback for trainees. Simulation also helps to emphasize the use of standardized, consistent technique, again confirming the need for a checklist-based approach.[11,36] Despite these data, most fellows are trained on continuing pregnancies.[37]

AMNIOCENTESIS: COMMON EDUCATIONAL PITFALLS

There are several common potential pitfalls with needle-based ultrasound procedures that trainees often fail to recognize (**Box 3**). First, the lateral and fundal aspects of the uterus have an ovoid shape, with the slope falling off rapidly as the edges are approached. Therefore, if a pocket is chosen at the far lateral aspect of the uterus, the needle can easily glide off the side, missing the uterus. For a similar reason, pockets of fluid should be visualized in 2 planes before any procedure. Pockets that appear adequate in the midsagittal plane can often be found to be narrow in the transverse plane, especially in the term amniocentesis, and therefore difficult to access (**Fig. 6**). During a reduction amniocentesis, if the pocket chosen is not central, the changing shape of the uterus as the fluid reduces can similarly result in the needle no longer being in the proper location. The operator must make an assessment of how the uterine shape will change as the procedure progresses.

The trainee is often unsure about the depth and direction of approach. This uncertainty can lead to the trainee being deeper than intended, and the tip can be lost at greater depths. Moving needles despite poor visualization is a common phenomenon noted in the simulation and education literature, and therefore the trainer must be aware of this common pitfall.[16] Marking the distance to traverse by ultrasound, and then discussing how much of the needle will be needed can help to

Box 3
Common amniocentesis pitfalls by trainees

1. Choosing a very lateral pocket
2. Failing to visualize pocket size in 2 planes
3. Failing to recognize how the pocket will change with withdrawal of fluid
4. Needle further advanced than realized
5. Choosing an approach too close to the ultrasound probe

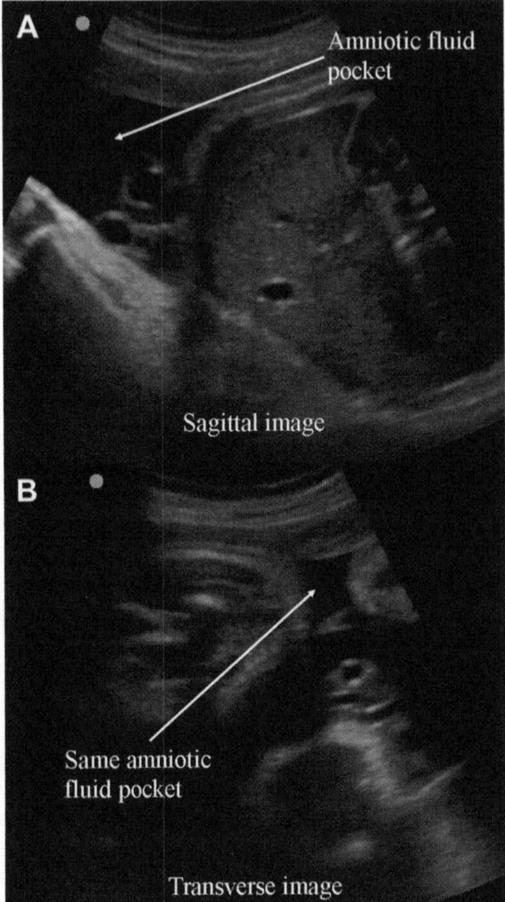

Fig. 6. Determining the approach requires visualization of the target pocket in 2 planes. Note that, although the fluid pocket assessed here appears adequate when viewed on midsagittal imaging (*A*), when it is viewed transversely (*B*) it is narrow and would be difficult to access. This condition is especially common with a term amniocentesis.

reduce this risk. However, advancing the needle too slowly can increase the risk of membrane tenting and uterine contraction, which are common reasons for failing to obtain fluid.[26]

The sonologist or training provider should also endeavor to keep the tip in view for the entire approach. Trainees often choose a site too close to the ultrasound probe when performing procedures, and inexperienced sonologists move the probe closer to the needle when failing to find the needle tip. Having the 2 objects closer together puts the sounds beams more parallel to the needle and makes visualization more difficult (**Fig. 7**, Videos 3 and 4). In addition, if the 2 objects are close together, this does not allow the sonographer or the physician to adjust in response to interference from the other operator. For most

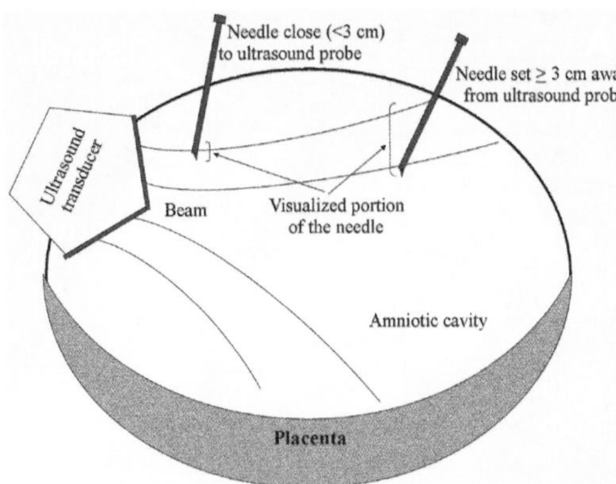

Fig. 7. Choice of distance from the ultrasound probe and needle visualization. Note that, as needle placement is closer to the ultrasound, but not in line, the visualized portion of the needle is smaller. Therefore, when doing an amniocentesis across the ultrasound beam, choosing a site farther from the needle and allowing the sonographic beam to be angled up at the needle improves visualization of the needle path.

approaches, having the probe at least 3 cm away and almost 45° inferior to the needle allows the maximum visualization of the needle and allows adjustment of the beam without interfering with the needle. This technique also naturally leads to a higher needle placement on the uterus, with the transducer lower, which is associated with less patient pain during the procedure.[38] In addition, looking away from the ultrasound screen and toward the patient's abdomen to assess the location and direction of both the needle and the ultrasound beam can eliminate many lost-needle moments.

FETAL BLOOD SAMPLING

FBS, also called percutaneous umbilical blood sampling starts in a manner similar to amniocentesis, so the general approach and discussion are the same, although the target is different. FBS is generally done to either directly access the fetal circulation to provide medications, blood, or platelet therapy, or to obtain fetal blood for testing. Because most mendelian genetic disorders can be tested from amniocytes, the genetic indications for FBS sampling are limited but include mosaic results on amniocentesis or CVS, as well as complex genetic disorders in which the specific mutation is not known.[26] Nongenetic indications for FBS include assessment for anemia, infection, and thrombocytopenia.[26]

The transducer should again be kept at least 3 cm from the needle to allow visualization of the length (see **Fig. 7**).[39] In general, either the umbilical vein just inside the umbilical cord placental insertion site to provide stability, or the fetal umbilical vein within the liver, are used for FBS and/or transfusion (**Fig. 8**). The discussion of which target is appropriate depends on many factors, including fetal position, samples needed, location of placenta and fetus, and preference of the operator. The intrahepatic approach has the advantage that any extravagated blood is reabsorbed within the abdominal cavity and therefore provides a depot of blood when there is ongoing fetal anemia. Studies of maternal serum α-fetoprotein before and after sampling suggest that there is significant mixing of the maternal and fetal components with any approach that transverses the placenta, and therefore this should be avoided if possible in patients in whom alloimmunization is a concern.[40]

Complications with FBS include streaming (generally self-limited), umbilical artery vasospasm, rupture of membranes, infection, or preterm labor, but can include fetal loss, especially in the already compromised fetus. Streaming rates are hard to estimate, but seem to be at least 30%, with bradycardias in at least 8%.[41] Loss rates are estimated be 1%, but estimates vary from 0% to 10%.[42] The best estimates suggest that the procedure is associated with an excess 1% to 2% loss rate per procedure, per patient, with significant variation by both operator experience and patient selection.[26] There seems to be a learning curve associated with the first 100 procedures, especially if the procedure is not regularly practiced.[39,40,43–45] The number of procedures that it takes to achieve mastery is higher than the

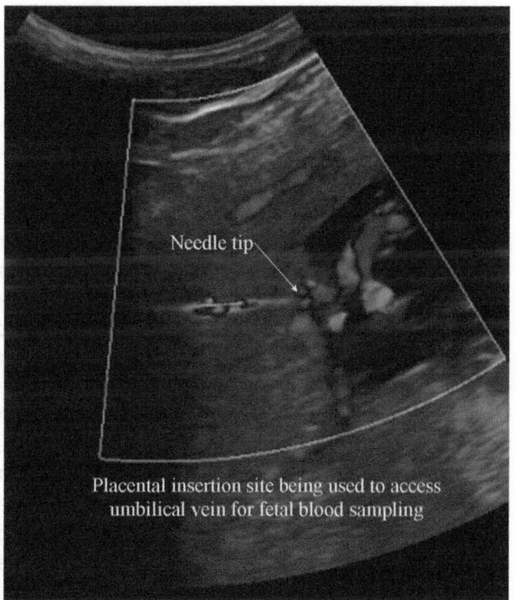

Fig. 8. FBS being performed within the umbilical vein just inside the umbilical cord insertion.

reported performance in fellowship by most graduates, in which the median reported number before graduation was only 5.[46] However, for fellows or trainees with direct supervision, the loss rate does not seem to be markedly increased compared with reported baseline risks.[44]

Because these are generally complex procedures with multiple steps, it is important that the team develop checklists and preprocedure stopchecks or huddles. These checks can help to ensure that all the needed personnel are present and aware of their roles in the procedure, and that all the needed equipment, sample transport containers, requisitions, blood products, and medications are present, appropriately administered, and accounted for. If opening and closing hematocrit or platelet counts will be needed, the appropriate laboratories need to be made aware of the procedure and be standing by to run samples. Given the complexity of these procedures, a checklist and specific roles for each team member are imperative, and allow learners to have a clear and consistent approach to the procedure. Simulation of these events, as well as complications that could occur during these events (such as fetal bradycardia or maternal vasovagal reaction), can help to find any systematic problems, which has been shown to be of value in other complex, team-based procedures.[10] Because most patients are not sedated before these procedures, being sure that all members of the team know their roles, as well as the terminology that will be used, is critical in maintaining patient confidence.

FBS: Simulation

Most specialists rarely perform FBS, because the indications for this procedure are decreasing with the widespread use of Rho(D) immunoglobulin and the large number of early screening options available. Simulation needs to a part of all programs that plan to credential in FBS before fellowship graduation given the limited numbers of procedures in most fellowships. There are currently no minimum numbers of procedures needed to credential in most programs, and no national standard, which is a phenomenon in other specialties as well.[47] In the only study to date, most maternal-fetal medicine fellows reported performing few procedures before graduation (fewer than 10), with 14% performing none and most (75%) thinking that they did not meet the minimum numbers needed for competency by their own standards.[46] Regardless, most fellows (86%) planned to perform FBS in practice.[46] Most concerning, among those planning to perform FBS in practice, 8% reported no formal training, 16% expected to graduate without performing a single procedure, and 71% did not think that they would meet the minimum number needed for competency.[46]

Simulation of FBS has been done with multiple different setups, and there is at least 1 commercially available simulator, with at least 1 other in development.[34] Simulation has also been reported on noncontinuing pregnancies.[19,45] Tongprasert and colleagues[41,48,49] completed a series of evaluations on skills after using a simulator created by filling an umbilical cord with synthetic blood, which was suspended within a water bath covered with a latex membrane or pig skin. A similar-looking, although less realistic, cord feel can also be achieved using an elongated balloon (**Fig. 9**). When practicing physicians who were trained with the simulator were compared with those who were not, use of the simulator was associated with an improvement in completion rate (94.8% vs 98.8%, $P = .011$) as well as an improved speed of completion (13.2 vs 6.4 minutes, $P<.001$) without a difference in loss rates.[49] In addition, among maternal-fetal medicine fellows who used this simulation method for 300 procedures before clinically independently performing FBS without direct supervision, the loss rate was 1.3%, which is consistent with reported loss data in practicing providers.[48] Skills seemed to plateau after completion of 60 procedures on ongoing pregnancies,[48] which is a much higher number for training than reported performance in fellowship by most graduates.[46]

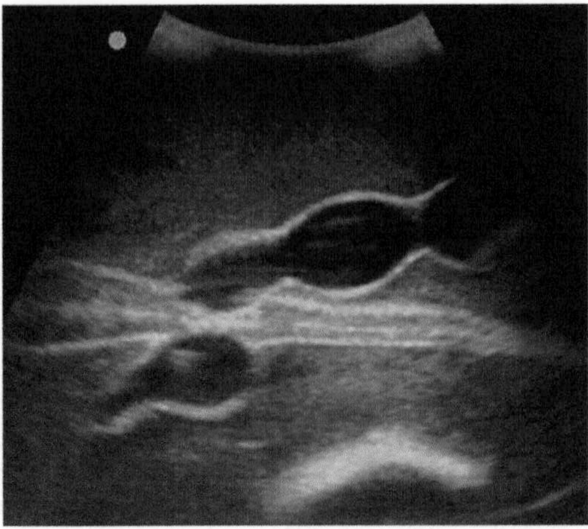

Fig. 9. Balloon FBS simulator. Elongated fluid-filled balloon suspended within a water bath, viewed through a gel pack for simulation of FBS. The size of the target can be varied with learner experience, and results in realistic streaming at the end of the attempt.

FBS: Common Educational Pitfalls

The educational pitfalls for FBS are similar to those described from amniocentesis, with a few additional concerns. Failure to have the appropriate paralytic medications available and already drawn up can result in losing access because of fetal movement. As noted with amniocentesis, learners have a tendency to be deeper than they realize, and this can result in a through-and-through penetration of the umbilical cord. Confirmation of intravascular placement, as well as transfusion flow, by Doppler can help to eliminate the placement of the needle into the abdomen or amniotic cavity.

CHORIONIC VILLUS SAMPLING

Because amniocentesis cannot safely be performed before 15 weeks, the primary use of CVS is to allow genetic testing of the fetus in the first trimester.[26] For many patients, obtaining detailed genetic information at an early age is critical to decision making while termination procedures are still readily available and before the increased risks of later pregnancy termination. Loss rates are approximately 1% higher than for amniocentesis (about 2.5%), partially because of the greater background miscarriage in the first 11 to 13 weeks of pregnancy. The most common complications with CVS include bleeding, with at least 7% to 10% of patients reporting procedure bleeding with a transcervical approach, and some spotting in up to one-third.[26] This complication occurs in less than 1% of transabdominal approaches.[26] Hematomas, infection, and rupture of membranes are the other most common complications, along with maternal cell contamination and failure to obtain adequate tissue.[26]

There is wide variation in the estimates of risk of loss after CVS. In addition to informing knowledge about loss rates, these trials also show the importance of training on CVS loss rates. The consensus on the large discrepancy in loss rates after CVS is that a large portion of this is caused by operator experience. The largest trial in the United States had an average of 325 cases per center and the Canadian trial had 106 cases per center, whereas the European trials had only 52 cases per center.[50–52] The loss rates from these trials correlate with this experience trend. Both the large Canadian randomized trial and the US nonrandomized trial did not show a difference in loss rates between amniocentesis and CVS, with loss rates of approximately 7% for all procedures (including chromosomal abnormalities and terminations of pregnancy).[50,51] In contrast, the European Medical Research Council showed that CVS had a 4.6% increased loss compared with amniocentesis.[52]

In addition, the US trial showed that number of passes required for an adequate sample is directly related to loss rates, with loss rates of 10.8% with 3 or more passes, and loss rates of 2.9% with 1 pass.[51] Based on these data, it seems that CVS has a prolonged learning curve, particularly the transcervical approach.[26] Some investigators have suggested that as many as 400 transabdominal procedures may be needed to achieve maximal safety, and the loss rates in trials that were repeated with successively more trained operators suggest this as well, with the most experienced operators having loss rates as low as 1.3% to 1.9%.[53–55] At least 1 large study suggests that fellows under direct supervision do not have a significantly higher loss rate; however, more than 300 procedures were performed by fellows, suggesting a high rate of exposure to procedures of trainees within this study.[56]

CVS: Credentialing

How many CVS procedures should be required before independent practice is not defined. Estimates range from 30 to 300, and this depends on route.[56–58] For transcervical CVS, most catheter companies require at least 25 procedures under direct supervision,[59] and, for most training programs, at least some of these must be performed on noncontinuing pregnancies. Other programs require a full 25 on noncontinuing pregnancies, followed by 25 under direct supervision. On the initiation of CVS training in the Netherlands, 50 training procedures were required, which was decreased to 30 and requirement to train on terminating pregnancies removed.[58] More rapid development of skills was associated with prior amniocentesis experience, and Wijnberger and colleagues[58] estimated that 175 procedures were needed to minimize risk, and therefore recommended that CVS training be centralized to a few centers to maximize proficiency. Even with training, continuous quality improvement with CVS improves outcomes.[56,57]

Despite the clear evidence of an extended learning curve, especially for transcervical CVS, most fellows are not receiving this degree of CVS training. Among surveyed fellows, although 82% of institutions performed CVS, only 53% of fellows had available training. Of these, 58% initiated training on terminating pregnancies, which means that 42% initiated training on continuing pregnancies without prior training. The median number of procedures was 3, with the median number of planned procedures before graduation being 40. Most (76%) thought that 50 or fewer procedures were needed for proficiency, and 88% thought that fewer than 70 were needed, despite the published estimates.[37,55,58] Of those trained, only 79% planned to continue CVS in practice; however, despite receiving no training, 16% of fellows planned to perform CVS in practice.[37]

CVS: Simulation

CVS training is limited and, therefore, to achieve the numbers recommended for safe performance of this skill, most clinicians are required to use a combination of both simulation, as well as performance under direct supervision. For simulation, there are no commercially available models, but there is a described simulator using cow or porcine heart.[17] Halved papayas prepared with 2 colors of layered gelatin and then wrapped with plastic wrap can be used to simulate the float of the catheter, as well as the aspiration technique. In addition, educational programs have been described that progress stepwise through needle and ultrasound-guided procedures from amniocentesis to transabdominal CVS to simple transcervical CVS to complex transvaginal CVS.[60]

For using the porcine model for transabdominal simulation, fixed or fresh placenta is placed within the hollowed-out heart over an internal balloon containing both water and a fetal pig. A second balloon is used to simulate the maternal bladder, and a needle is passed into the placenta under ultrasound visualization.[17] This model can also be placed within an artificial pelvis. An artificial os is then created in the apex of the cow heart to simulate a transvaginal approach.[17] In a study of 23 maternal-fetal medicine attendings and 8 fellows, 100% thought that these simulators could be used to teach fellows and staff. In addition, the look on ultrasound was deemed realistic by 87% of faculty and 86% of fellows, and 77% of the faculty and 88% of the fellows thought that the passage of the needle on the transabdominal passage was realistic.[17] Most planned to use these simulators, and would be willing to buy them to use with faculty and fellows. The negative comments on this simulation method were related to the feel of the placenta, which was fixed and therefore stiff; fresh placenta improved both the appearance and haptic feedback.[17] Recently a model for CVS simulation using tofu, beans and chicken breast has also been described, with good haptic feedback, ability to aspirate tofu "villi" and minimal degradation after multiple users and passes.[61]

CVS: Common Educational Pitfalls

For CVS performed abdominally, the approach and preparation are similar to those of amniocentesis, except that the target is a full-length pass into the long axis of the placenta (Video 5), avoiding the amniotic cavity. The trainee and clinician should discuss the approach with the additional understanding that the uterus is more reactive to stimuli in the first trimester and may acutely change shape or undergo a focal contraction as the needle is placed, distorting the approach. Therefore, readjustment is often needed during these procedures and, to be prepared, the trainee and supervising clinician should discuss the approach and how the uterus is likely to change in shape. The uterus is small, and planning the relationship of the ultrasound transducer to the location of the needle to allow change in the approach as the procedure progresses is critical. As with an amniocentesis, using a simulated needle can aid with this planning.

For the CVS performed transcervically, the preprocedure planning between the trainee and teacher is of the upmost importance, because the guiding physician cannot easily adjust or change the planned approach once the procedure is initiated. To perform a CVS with a minimal risk of complications, the physician who will be performing the procedure must make an assessment of the full length of the placenta and its relationship to the cervical os.[26] In addition, focal uterine contractions, common at this gestational age, distort the uterine position and can make it difficult to find a safe path for the catheter. The trainee may not realize that waiting for these to resolve (which can take as long as 60 minutes) can improve the visualization.[26] The bladder is typically filled to manipulate the uterine position; however, the trainee may fail to recognize when the bladder is overdistended, resulting in elevation of the uterus out of the pelvis. This elevation both elongates the vagina, making cervical visualization with the speculum more difficult, and lengthens the sampling path, preventing the catheter from being manipulated as easily.[26]

The trainee should know the position of the catheter at all times within the uterine cavity. When sampling transcervically, there is a moment when the catheter is not visible beneath the metal shadow of the speculum (**Fig. 10**, see Video 6). The trainee should have a feel of the internal os, float the catheter to this point, and then wait to be found by the guiding sonographer or clinician. The internal cervical os may not be directly in line with the presumed midline path initially delineated while planning, and redirection may be needed at this point. The trainee also should not advance the catheter beyond this point without direct visualization, and, as with amniocentesis, trainees may have a tendency to advance without visualization. If a curve is placed into the catheter (which is generally needed), the notch on the handle should

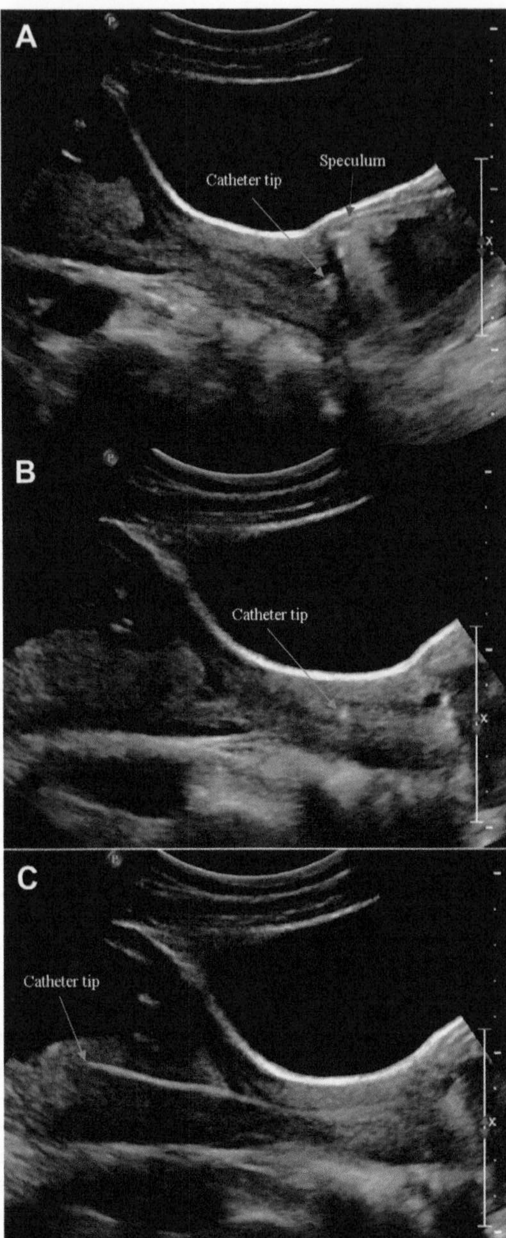

Fig. 10. Transcervical CVS catheter passage. During the performance of a transcervical CVS, the catheter is not visible while under the shadow of the speculum. As the tip passes, it becomes visible past the shadow of the speculum (*A*) and comes more into view as it moves into the plane of the transducer (*B, C*). Also note how elongated the cervix is with a full bladder (*C*), as well as how the bladder moves the uterus and placenta in a straight-line access. The trainee may fail to recognize that, if this is underfilled or becomes overdistended, the CVS will become more difficult.

be used in a consistent manner, in line with the curve (ie, the curve either goes directly toward or away from this notch) so that this will provide a visual cue to the direction of the curve within the uterus. In addition, if the curve needs to be changed to posterior, the catheter will need to be placed through the cervix with the curve anterior, then flipped once just past the internal os. This situation results in loss of the tip of the catheter with shadowing, so the operating trainee and the guiding sonographer need be aware of this, and find the tip as it moves back into plane.

SUMMARY

Training for ultrasound procedures has considerable variability in the approach and methodologies used. Most ultrasound-based procedures are still taught using a traditional apprenticeship method of training; however, to allow for the conflicting interests of both patient safety and the training of future physicians, procedural training must include some combination of didactic training, observation, simulation, and performance in a monitored setting. Creation of standardized approaches and stepwise training methodologies may also help to reduce complications and improve training.

SUPPLEMENTARY DATA

Videos related to this article can be found online at doi:http://dx.doi.org/10.1016/j.cult.2012.08.017.

REFERENCES

1. Magee D, Zhu Y, Ratnalingam R, et al. An augmented reality simulator for ultrasound guided needle placement training. Med Biol Eng Comput 2007;45:957–67.
2. Tafra L. The learning curve and sentinel node biopsy. Am J Surg 2001;182:347–50.
3. Blessed WB, Lacoste H, Welch RA. Obstetrician-gynecologists performing genetic amniocentesis may be misleading themselves and their patients. Am J Obstet Gynecol 2001;184:1340–2 [discussion: 42–4].
4. Chenkin J, Lee S, Huynh T, et al. Procedures can be learned on the Web: a randomized study of ultrasound-guided vascular access training. Acad Emerg Med 2008;15:949–54.
5. Xeroulis GJ, Park J, Moulton CA, et al. Teaching suturing and knot-tying skills to medical students: a randomized controlled study comparing computer-based video instruction and (concurrent and summary) expert feedback. Surgery 2007;141:442–9.
6. Moulton CA, Dubrowski A, Macrae H, et al. Teaching surgical skills: what kind of practice makes perfect?: a randomized, controlled trial. Ann Surg 2006;244:400–9.
7. Moulton CA, Regehr G, Lingard L, et al. Operating from the other side of the table: control dynamics and the surgeon educator. J Am Coll Surg 2010;210:79–86.
8. Moulton CA, Regehr G, Lingard L, et al. 'Slowing down when you should': initiators and influences of the transition from the routine to the effortful. J Gastrointest Surg 2010;14:1019–26.
9. Moulton CA, Regehr G, Lingard L, et al. Slowing down to stay out of trouble in the operating room: remaining attentive in automaticity. Acad Med 2010;85:1571–7.
10. Nishisaki A, Nguyen J, Colborn S, et al. Evaluation of multidisciplinary simulation training on clinical performance and team behavior during tracheal intubation procedures in a pediatric intensive care unit. Pediatr Crit Care Med 2011;12:406–14.
11. Berenholtz SM, Pronovost PJ, Lipsett PA, et al. Eliminating catheter-related bloodstream infections in the intensive care unit. Crit Care Med 2004;32:2014–20.
12. Timor-Tritsch IE, Yeh MN. In vitro training model for diagnostic and therapeutic fetal intravascular needle puncture. Am J Obstet Gynecol 1987;157:858–9.
13. Maher JE, Kleinman GE, Lile W, et al. The construction and utility of an amniocentesis trainer. Am J Obstet Gynecol 1998;179:1225–7.
14. Smith JF Jr, Bergmann M, Gildersleeve R, et al. A simple model for learning stereotactic skills in ultrasound-guided amniocentesis. Obstet Gynecol 1998;92:303–5.
15. Zubair I, Marcotte MP, Weinstein L, et al. A novel amniocentesis model for learning stereotactic skills. Am J Obstet Gynecol 2006;194:846–8.
16. Sites BD, Gallagher JD, Cravero J, et al. The learning curve associated with a simulated ultrasound-guided interventional task by inexperienced anesthesia residents. Reg Anesth Pain Med 2004;29:544–8.
17. McWeeney DT, Schwendemann WD, Nitsche JF, et al. Transabdominal and transcervical chorionic villus sampling models to teach maternal-fetal medicine fellows. Am J Perinatol 2012;29(7):497–502.
18. Grace D, Thornburg L, Gray A, et al. Characteristics of women who consent to a training invasive prenatal procedure during second-trimester termination of pregnancy. Am J Obstet Gynecol 2007;197:S184.
19. Thornburg L, Grace D, Gray A, et al. Training for second-trimester invasive pregnancy procedures in a maternal-fetal medicine fellowship. Am J Obstet Gynecol 2007;197:S185.
20. Ward RH, Modell B, Petrou M, et al. Method of sampling chorionic villi in first trimester of pregnancy under guidance of real time ultrasound. BMJ 1983;286:1542–4.
21. Seeds JW. Diagnostic mid trimester amniocentesis: how safe? Am J Obstet Gynecol 2004;191:607–15.

22. Silver RK, Russell TL, Kambich MP, et al. Midtrimester amniocentesis. Influence of operator caseload on sampling efficiency. J Reprod Med 1998;43:191–5.
23. Tabor A, Alfirevic Z. Update on procedure-related risks for prenatal diagnosis techniques. Fetal Diagn Ther 2010;27:1–7.
24. Midtrimester amniocentesis for prenatal diagnosis. Safety and accuracy. JAMA 1976;236:1471–6.
25. Randomised trial to assess safety and fetal outcome of early and midtrimester amniocentesis. The Canadian Early and Mid-trimester Amniocentesis Trial (CEMAT) Group. Lancet 1998;351:242–7.
26. Wapner RJ, Jenkins T, Khalek N. Prenatal diagnosis of congenital disorders. In: Creasy RK, Resnik R, Iams JD, editors. Creasy and Resnik's maternal-fetal medicine: principles and practice. Philadelphia: Saunders/Elsevier; 2009.
27. Wilson RD, Langlois S, Johnson JA. Mid-trimester amniocentesis fetal loss rate. J Obstet Gynaecol Can 2007;29:586–95.
28. Eddleman KA, Malone FD, Sullivan L, et al. Pregnancy loss rates after midtrimester amniocentesis. Obstet Gynecol 2006;108:1067–72.
29. ACOG Committee on Practice Bulletins. ACOG practice bulletin no. 77: screening for fetal chromosomal abnormalities. Obstet Gynecol 2007;109:217–27.
30. Sonek J, Nicolaides K, Sadowsky G, et al. Articulated needle guide: report on the first 30 cases. Obstet Gynecol 1989;74:821–3.
31. Pittini R, Oepkes D, Macrury K, et al. Teaching invasive perinatal procedures: assessment of a high fidelity simulator-based curriculum. Ultrasound Obstet Gynecol 2002;19:478–83.
32. Nitsche JF, McWeeney DT, Schwendemann WD, et al. In-utero stenting: development of a low-cost high-fidelity task trainer. Ultrasound Obstet Gynecol 2009;34:720–3.
33. Blue Phantom amniocentesis ultrasound training model. 2012. Available at: http://www.bluephantom.com/product/Amniocentesis-Ultrasound-Training-Model.aspx?cid=429. Accessed September 9, 2012.
34. Limbs and Things cordocentesis trainer. 2012. Available at: http://limbsandthings.com/us/products/cordocentesis-trainer/. Accessed September 9, 2012.
35. Nizard J, Duyme M, Ville Y. Teaching ultrasound-guided invasive procedures in fetal medicine: learning curves with and without an electronic guidance system. Ultrasound Obstet Gynecol 2002;19:274–7.
36. Nizard J. Amniocentesis: technique and education. Curr Opin Obstet Gynecol 2010;22:152–4.
37. Jenkins TM, Sciscione AC, Wapner RJ, et al. Training in chorionic villus sampling: limited experience for US fellows. Am J Obstet Gynecol 2004;191:1288–90.
38. Harris A, Monga M, Wicklund CA, et al. Clinical correlates of pain with amniocentesis. Am J Obstet Gynecol 2004;191:542–5.
39. Ville Y, Cooper M, Revel A, et al. Development of a training model for ultrasound-guided invasive procedures in fetal medicine. Ultrasound Obstet Gynecol 1995;5:180–3.
40. Weiner C, Grant S, Hudson J, et al. Effect of diagnostic and therapeutic cordocentesis on maternal serum alpha-fetoprotein concentration. Am J Obstet Gynecol 1989;161:706–8.
41. Tongprasert F, Tongsong T, Wanapirak C, et al. Experience of the first 50 cases of cordocentesis after training with model. J Med Assoc Thai 2005;88:728–33.
42. Ghidini A, Sepulveda W, Lockwood CJ, et al. Complications of fetal blood sampling. Am J Obstet Gynecol 1993;168:1339–44.
43. Nicolaides KH, Soothill PW, Rodeck CH, et al. Ultrasound-guided sampling of umbilical cord and placental blood to assess fetal wellbeing. Lancet 1986;1:1065–7.
44. Perry KG Jr, Hess LW, Roberts WE, et al. Cordocentesis (funipuncture) by maternal-fetal fellows: the learning curve. Fetal Diagn Ther 1991;6:87–92.
45. Daffos F, Capella-Pavlovsky M, Forestier F. Fetal blood sampling via the umbilical cord using a needle guided by ultrasound. Report of 66 cases. Prenat Diagn 1983;3:271–7.
46. Grace D, Thornburg LL, Grey A, et al. Training for percutaneous umbilical blood sampling during Maternal Fetal Medicine fellowship in the United States. Prenat Diagn 2009;29:790–3.
47. Berns JS, O'Neill WC. Performance of procedures by nephrologists and nephrology fellows at U.S. nephrology training programs. Clin J Am Soc Nephrol 2008;3:941–7.
48. Tongprasert F, Srisupundit K, Luewan S, et al. Midpregnancy cordocentesis training of maternal-fetal medicine fellows. Ultrasound Obstet Gynecol 2010;36:65–8.
49. Tongprasert F, Wanapirak C, Sirichotiyakul S, et al. Training in cordocentesis: the first 50 case experience with and without a cordocentesis training model. Prenat Diagn 2010;30:467–70.
50. Multicentre randomised clinical trial of chorion villus sampling and amniocentesis. First report. Canadian Collaborative CVS-Amniocentesis Clinical Trial Group. Lancet 1989;1:1–6.
51. Rhoads GG, Jackson LG, Schlesselman SE, et al. The safety and efficacy of chorionic villus sampling for early prenatal diagnosis of cytogenetic abnormalities. N Engl J Med 1989;320:609–17.
52. Medical Research Council European trial of chorion villus sampling. MRC working party on the evaluation of chorion villus sampling. Lancet 1991;337:1491–9.
53. Philip J, Silver RK, Wilson RD, et al. Late first-trimester invasive prenatal diagnosis: results of an international randomized trial. Obstet Gynecol 2004;103:1164–73.
54. Caughey AB, Hopkins LM, Norton ME. Chorionic villus sampling compared with amniocentesis and

the difference in the rate of pregnancy loss. Obstet Gynecol 2006;108:612–6.

55. Saura R, Gauthier B, Taine L, et al. Operator experience and fetal loss rate in transabdominal CVS. Prenat Diagn 1994;14:70–1.
56. Chueh JT, Goldberg JD, Wohlferd MM, et al. Comparison of transcervical and transabdominal chorionic villus sampling loss rates in nine thousand cases from a single center. Am J Obstet Gynecol 1995;173:1277–82.
57. Boehm FH, Salyer SL, Dev VG, et al. Chorionic villus sampling: quality control–a continuous improvement model. Am J Obstet Gynecol 1993;168:1766–75.
58. Wijnberger LD, van der Schouw YT, Christiaens GC. Learning in medicine: chorionic villus sampling. Prenat Diagn 2000;20:241–6.
59. Training requirements for physicians using the Cook® chorionic villus sampling set. Available at: http://www.cookmedical.com/wh/content/mmedia/WH-SF-CVS-EN-0708.pdf. Accessed June 21, 2012.
60. Isada NB, Johnson MP, Pryde PG, et al. Technical aspects of transcervical chorionic villus sampling. Fetal Diagn Ther 1994;9:19–28.
61. Wax J, Cartin A, Pinette M. The birds and the beans: a low-fidelity simulator for chorionic villus sampling skill acquisition. J Ultrasound Med 2012;31:1271–5.

Index

Note: Page numbers of article titles are in **boldface** type.

A

Abdominal wall defects, **55–67**
  bladder exstrophy, 56, 58, 60–61, 64
  cloacal exstrophy, 56–58, 60–61, 64
  ectopia cordis (pentalogy of Cantrell), 56, 59–60, 64
  embryology of, 55
  gastroschisis, 55–57, 59–65
  incidence of, 55
  limb-body wall complex, 56, 58–59, 61, 64
  omphalocele, 56–57, 60–65
  ultrasound for
    bowel appearance, 60, 63–64
    extracorporeal organs, 60
    limiting membrane in, 59–61
    malformations associated with, 60, 63–64
    umbilical cord insertion, 60–62
Achondrogenesis, 33
Achondroplasia, 33
Alloimmunization, anemia in, 79–80
Amniocentesis
  for anemia, 82–83
  training for, 92–96
Anemia, fetal, **79–87**
  causes of, 79–81
  delivery planning in, 84
  history of, 79
  pearls and pitfalls in, 82–85
  treatment of, 82–85
  ultrasound for, 81–82
Aneuploidy
  screening for, in obesity, 41–43
  ventriculomegaly in, 15–16
Aqueduct of Sylvius obstruction, ventriculomegaly in, 14
Aqueductal stenosis, ventriculomegaly in, 14–16
Arteriovenous malformations, anemia in, 82
Ascites
  in abdominal wall defects, 59, 61
  in congenital cystic adenomatoid malformation, 50–51
  in hydronephrosis, 72, 76

B

Beckwith-Wiedemann syndrome, 57, 64
Bladder exstrophy, 56, 58, 60–61, 64
Blood sampling
  in anemia, 83–85
  training for, 96–98
Bowel appearance, in abdominal wall defects, 60, 63–64
Bronchogenic cysts, 53
Bronchopulmonary sequestration, 52–53

C

Calicectasis, 72
Campomelic dysplasia, 33
Cardiac anomalies
  in abdominal wall defects, 63–64
  screening for, in obesity, 43–45
Cardiofemoral index, in anemia, 82
Cephalocentesis, for ventriculomegaly, 20, 22
Cerclage, cervical length measurement and, 4, 6, 8–9
Cervical length.measurement, **1–11**
  challenges in, 2–3
  digital method for, 1
  implications of decreased length and, 5
  in asymptomatic patients, 8–9
  in low-risk patients, 8–9
  technique for, 1–3
  timing of, 4
  with history of preterm birth, 5–6
  with symptoms of preterm labor, 6–7
Cervical pregnancy, versus cesarean scar ectopic pregnancy, 29
Cesarean scar ectopic pregnancy, **27–30**
Chorioangiomas, anemia in, 82
Chorionic villus sampling, training for, 98–101
Cloacal exstrophy, 56–58, 60–61, 64
COL1A gene mutations, in skeletal dysplasias, 35
Color Doppler evaluation, for bronchopulmonary sequestration, 52
Congenital anomalies of the kidney and urinary tract, 70–71
Congenital cystic adenomatoid malformation, 49–52
Congenital high airway obstruction, 53
Congenital lobar inflation, 53
Corticosteroids
  for anemia, 84
  for congenital cystic adenomatoid malformation, 51
Curved cervix, 2
Cyst(s)
  bronchogenic, 53
  neurenteric, 53
  umbilical cord, 65
Cystic adenomatoid malformation, congenital, 49–52

Ultrasound Clin 8 (2013) 105–108
http://dx.doi.org/10.1016/S1556-858X(12)00124-7

D

Doppler evaluation. *See also* Color Doppler evaluation.
- for anemia, 80–85
- for cesarean scar ectopic pregnancy, 28
- for fetomaternal hemorrhage, 80

Double collecting systems, in kidney, 72
Down syndrome
- hydronephrosis and, 73, 75
- ventriculomegaly and, 16

Dyserythropoioetic anemia, 81

E

Ectopia cordis (pentalogy of Cantrell), 56, 59–60, 64
Ectopic pregnancy, in cesarean scar, **27–30**
Ectopic ureter, 71–72
Epispadias, 56–58, 60–61, 64
Exstropy-epispadias complex disorders, 56–58, 60–61, 64
Extracorporeal organs, in abdominal wall defects, 60
Extralobar bronchopulmonary sequestration, 52

F

FaSTER (First and Second Trimester Screening) trial, 41–43
Fetal abdominal wall defects, **55–67**
Fetal anemia, **79–87**
Fetal fibronectin testing, for preterm labor detection, 6–7
Fetal hydronephrosis, **69–77**
Fetal lung masses, **49–54**
Fetal ventriculomegaly, **13–25**
Fetal weight, estimation of, in obesity, 45–46
Fetomaternal hemorrhage, anemia in, 80
FGFR3 gene mutations, in skeletal dysplasias, 34–35
Fibronectin testing, for preterm labor detection, 6–7
First and Second Trimester Screening (FaSTER) trial, 41–43
Funneling, in cervical length measurement, 2–3

G

Gastroschisis, 55–57, 59–65
Genetic disorders
- screening for, in obesity, 42–45
- ventriculomegaly in, 14–16

Gestational adjusted prediction method, 46
Gestational sac, bulging of, in cesarean scar ectopic pregnancy, 28
Glucose-6-phosphate dehydrogenase deficiency, anemia in, 81

H

Hadlock formula, for fetal growth restriction, 64
Heart, ultrasound for, in anemia, 82
Hemoglobinopathies, anemia in, 80
Hemolytic crisis, in hemoglobinopathies, 81
Hemorrhage, fetal, anemia in, 80
Herniation
- midgut, 65
- umbilical, 65

Hydrocephalus
- as cause of ventriculomegaly, 14–16
- definition of, 14

Hydronephrosis, **69–77**
- bilateral, 73
- definition of, 69
- Down syndrome and, 73
- embryology of, 69–70
- etiology of, 71–73
- transient, 71
- treatment of, 73–74
- ultrasound for, 70–71, 74–76

Hydrops fetalis
- in anemia, **79–87**
- in bronchopulmonary sequestration, 52
- in congenital cystic adenomatoid malformation, 50–51

I

Immunoglobulin G, intravenous, for anemia, 84
Infections
- anemia in, 80
- ventriculomegaly in, 15–16

Intralobar bronchopulmonary sequestration, 52
Intraperitoneal transfusion, for anemia, 84

J

Jarco-Levin syndrome, 33

K

Kidney
- dysplasia of, 72
- hydronephrosis of, **69–77**

L

Laryngeal atresia (congenital high airway obstruction), 53
LeCAM gene mutations, ventriculomegaly in, 14–16
Limb-body wall complex, 56, 58–59, 61, 64
Limiting membranes, in abdominal wall defects, 59–61
Liver, in omphalocele, 57, 62–63
Lobar inflation, congenital, 53
Lower urinary tract obstruction, 71–76
Lung masses, fetal, ultrasound for, **49–54**
- bronchopulmonary sequestration, 52–53
- congenital cystic adenomatoid malformation, 49–52
- congenital high airway obstruction, 53

M

Macrocystic cystic adenomatoid malformation, congenital, 50
Macrosomia, prediction of, 45–46
Magnetic resonance imaging
for bronchopulmonary sequestration, 52
for congenital cystic adenomatoid malformation, 50–51
for ventriculomegaly, 20
Malformations, n abdominal wall defects, 60, 63–64
Megacystis, 72
Megacystis-microcolon-intestinal hypoperistalsis, 71, 73–74
Megaureter, 71–74
Microcolon, 73
Microcystic cystic adenomatoid malformation, congenital, 50
Middle cerebral artery Doppler peak systolic velocity, in anemia, 80–81
Midgut herniation, 65
Mineralization, defects of, in skeletal dysplasias, 32–33
Miscarriage, spontaneous, versus cesarean scar ectopic pregnancy, 29
Multicystic dysplastic kidney, 71–72
Myometrium, defects in, in cesarean scar ectopic pregnancy, 28

N

Neural tube defects, screening for, in obesity, 43
Neurenteric cysts, 53
Neurodevelopmental outcome, in ventriculomegaly, 19–20
Nuchal translucency measurement, in obesity, 41–42

O

Obesity, **39–47**
prevalence of, 39
ultrasound for, 39–41
fetal weight estimation in, 45–46
first-trimester, 41–42
second-trimester, 42–45
timing of, 44–45
Obstetric ultrasound
for abdominal wall defects, **55–67**
for cervical length measurement, **1–11**
for cesarean scar ectopic pregnancy, **27–30**
for fetal anemia, **79–87**
for fetal hydronephrosis, **69–77**
for fetal lung masses, **49–54**
for fetal skeletal dysplasia, **31–38**
for fetal ventriculomegaly, **13–25**
obesity effects on, **39–47**
training for, **89–103**
Ohio State University protocol, for cervical length measurement, 6–7
Oligohydramnios, in hydronephrosis, 70–76
Omphalocele, 56–57, 60–65
Osteochondrodysplasias. *See* Skeletal dysplasias.
Osteogenesis imperfecta, 33, 37

P

Parvovirus infections, anemia in, 80
Pelviectasis, 72
Pentalogy of Cantrell (ectopia cordis), 56, 59–60, 64
Percutaneous umbilical blood sampling
in anemia, 83–85
training for, 96–98
Pericardial effusion, in congenital cystic adenomatoid malformation, 50–51
Phenobarbital, for anemia, 84
Placenta, malformation of, anemia in, 82
Placenta accreta, versus cesarean scar ectopic pregnancy, 29–30
Plasmapheresis, for anemia, 84
Polyhydramnios, in congenital cystic adenomatoid malformation, 50–51
Posterior urethral valves, 71–72, 74
Preterm labor and birth, cervical length measurement in, 5–7
Progesterone supplementation, cervical length measurement and, 4, 6, 8–9
Prune-belly syndrome, 71, 73–74
Pulmonary dysplasia, in hydronephrosis, 72
Pulmonary hypoplasia, in congenital cystic adenomatoid malformation, 51
Pyeletasis, 70, 74

R

Renal pelvic diameter, in hydronephrosis, 70–71
Rh antibodies, anemia due to, 79–80

S

Skeletal dysplasias, **31–38**
classification of, 31
developmental aspects of, 32
pathophysiology of, 34–33, 37
prevalence of, 31
referral in, 36
ultrasound findings in, 32–36
Skin edema, in congenital cystic adenomatoid malformation, 50–51
Sliding organ sign, in cesarean scar ectopic pregnancy, 29
Society of Fetal Urology criteria, for hydronephrosis, 70

T

Thalassemia, anemia in, 80–81
Thanatophoric dysplasia, 33, 36
Thoracentesis
for bronchopulmonary sequestration, 52
for congenital cystic adenomatoid malformation, 51
Thoraco-abdominal syndrome (Pentalogy of Cantrell), 56, 59–60, 64
Thoracoamniotic shunting
for bronchopulmonary sequestration, 52
for congenital cystic adenomatoid malformation, 51
Three-dimentional ultrasound
for cesarean scar ectopic pregnancy, 28–29
for ventriculomegaly, 18–19
Training, for ultrasound procedures, **89–103**
approaches to, 91–92
didactic knowledge in, 89–90
for amniocentesis, 92–96
for chorionic villus sampling, 98–101
for fetal blood sampling, 96–98
planning in, 90–91
simulation, 91–92
Transfusions, for anemia, 80–81
Transperineal ultrasound, for cervical length measurement, 1–2
Transvaginal ultrasound
for cervical length measurement, 1–3
for cesarean scar ectopic pregnancy, **27–30**
Trisomy 21
hydronephrosis and, 73, 75
ventriculomegaly in, 16
Twin-twin transfusion syndrome, anemia in, 80

U

Umbilical cord
herniation at, 65
insertion abnormalities of, in abdominal wall defects, 60–62
transfusion through, 83–84
Ureter
dilated (megaureter), 71–74
ectopic, 71–72
Ureteroceles, 71–72, 74
Ureteropelvic junction obstruction, 71–74
Urethra
atresia of, 71, 73
exstrophy of, 58
Urinary tract, embryology of, 69–70
Urinomas, 74

V

Ventriculomegaly, **13–25**
anatomy of, 16
causes of, 14–16
counseling on, 20
definition of, 13–14
diagnosis of, 14
embryology of, 16
incidence of, 13
long-term outcome of, 19–20
magnetic resonance imaging for, 20
mortality risk in, 19–20
regression of, 20
treatment of, 20
ultrasound technique for, 16–18, 21
variants of, 21
Vesicoamniotic shunt, for hydronephrosis, 76
Vesicoureteral reflux, 71–73
Viral infections, anemia in, 80

W

Weight, fetal, estimation of, in obesity, 45–46

X

Xerocytosis, 81

Printed and bound by CPI Group (UK) Ltd, Croydon, CR0 4YY
03/10/2024
01040332-0010